FOREWORD BY **William Davis, MD**, AUTHOR OF ***Wheat Belly***

INTRODUCTION by **Mark Sisson**, AUTHOR OF ***The Primal Blueprint***

RICH FOOD

POOR FOOD

THE ULTIMATE **GROCERY PURCHASING SYSTEM** (GPS)

Shop Smart, Shop Healthy
Save Time, Save Money
Avoid Hype and
Harmful Ingredients

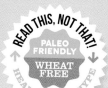

JAYSON CALTON, PhD AND MIRA CALTON, CN

PRIMAL BLUEPRINT PUBLISHING

D0052871

RICH FOOD, POOR FOOD

Library of Congress Control Number: 2013930098

Library of Congress Cataloging-in-Publication Data is on file with the publisher

Calton, Mira 1971- ; and Calton, Jayson, 1971-

Rich Food, Poor Food: The Ultimate Grocery Purchasing System / Mira Calton, CN, and Jayson Calton, PhD

ISBN: 9780984755172

1. Diet   2. Health   3. Weight Loss

Copy Editor: Tara VanTimmeren, Jessica Taylor Tudzin

Index: Gail Kearns, Jessica Taylor Tudzin

Cover Photography: Sara Hanna Photography

Cover Design: Janée Meadows

Publisher: Primal Blueprint Publishing. 23805 Stuart Ranch Rd. Suite 145 Malibu, CA 90265

For information on quantity discounts, please call 888-774-6259 or visit primalbluperintpublishing.com

WE DEDICATE THIS BOOK *to the incredible men and women who work tirelessly each day, often without recognition, to supply us with high-quality Rich Foods, and to our readers, who are dedicated to the importance of these treasures.*

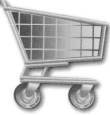

Contents

Foreword

If you are among the nutritionally inquisitive, enough to pick up this wonderful book written by Mira and Jayson Calton, then you likely already know a few things about proteins, fats, and carbohydrates, the macronutrients in our diet.

But what about *micro*nutrients? They may be found in much smaller quantities, thus the "micro-" designation—but don't let size fool you! Despite being present in milligram or microgram quantities, i.e., *a thousandth or millionth of a gram,* compared with the thousand- or million-fold greater gram quantities of macronutrients, micronutrients are just as necessary to health and life. Micronutrients are a much forgotten component of food, neglected in many discussions of nutrition yet as critical as any macronutrient.

We often talk about cutting or increasing this or that macronutrient, such as cutting carbohydrates or increasing fat. But we virtually never have to talk about cutting our micronutrients, since most of us struggle to even achieve the small but crucial quantities we need! *Rich Food, Poor Food* reminds us that there is an enormously powerful world of micronutrients that exist in parallel to our need for macronutrients. Mind only your macronutrients but neglect your micronutrients, and you may still be disappointed in the weight loss and health effects. Pay attention to the world of micronutrients, and you may be rewarded by the compound benefits of both worlds.

Once you are familiar with the issues raised by the Caltons, you will be talking the language of micronutrients, talking about the healthy and rich sources of selenium, iodine, and phylloquinone in the Rich Foods that you enjoy! The Caltons also discuss the issue closest and dearest to me, the dangers of "healthy whole grains," discussing how and why wheat—this Poor Food that has come to dominate our modern diets, is in reality the corrupt and destructive product of genetics research that should be eaten by no human.

In *Rich Food, Poor Food,* the Caltons educate, delight, and tantalize readers with their straight-shooting "here are the facts" style. Short of actually showing up at your front door and taking your hand down the aisle of the farmers market or grocery store, the Caltons show you, step by step, inch by inch, and micronutrient by micronutrient, how to best accomplish a healthy diet and lifestyle rich with the health benefits of plentiful micronutrients.

William Davis, MD
Author, #1 *New York Times* Bestseller, *Wheat Belly*

Acknowledgments

We want to thank Mark Sisson, our publisher, for seeing the true potential of this book and swooping in at the eleventh hour to help guide and direct us to completion. Thank you for bringing your invaluable insight to the table and allowing us the creative license to make this guide come alive. We would also like to thank our first publishers, Francesca and Ellen; without your early vision, *Naked Calories* and *Rich Food, Poor Food* may never have been possible. We can't say enough about how much fun Michele brings to the editing table. She cleans up our words, and in turn, those words have cleaned up her pantry. Apologies to her husband and children, who have watched as the sugar and wheat mysteriously disappeared—you'll thank us one day. To Lisa, you may have come to the game late, but you have hit a home run designing this guide. You added pop to our pronouns and color to our callouts. To our literary agent, Beth, thank you so much for riding this roller coaster with us; the value of your guidance is immeasurable and your blatant honesty refreshing. A special thanks to Bill Davis, MD, for taking the time to write our foreword. We hope our book will add to the incredible work you have already done—helping millions to discover health through the elimination of Poor Foods. To Brad and the entire Primal Team, thank you for viewing with fresh eyes and ideas. To our friends and family, both live and on Facebook, we thank you for your support, suggestions, and words of encouragement. To our ranchers, Kathy and Steve, chef Al Rosas of the Organic Chef Foods, and to everyone at the O'Brien Family Farm, without all of you, our fridge would be bare and our dog would be hungry. Thank you for supplying us with truly Rich Food. And last, but certainly not least, to the many Rich Food manufacturers who got involved with this project—thank you! Together we will continue to change the world.

"Ever feel like navigating your local supermarket involves a frustrating obstacle course fraught with confusing labels and misleading claims? Rich Food, Poor Food gives you everything you need to know to make smart, nutrient-rich food choices that save you time, money, and your health. Don't step into another grocery store without it!"

—JJ Virgin, CNS, CHFI, author of *The Virgin Diet*

"As a holistic nutritionist, I work with clients every day who are ready to make better food choices, but the grocery store remains a minefield of edible food-like products that leaves them flat-out frustrated. In Rich Food, Poor Food, Mira and Jayson Calton demystify the grocery store aisles by directing you to exactly which products they want you to buy and teach you why those are your best bets. Their GPS (Grocery Purchasing System) is a nearly foolproof way to navigate through any store to find which items will deliver the most nutrient-bang for your buck. If you're tired of the confusion caused by media hype about the latest 'health foods,' grab a copy of this book and hit the stores—you'll be armed for battle and come out a nutritional winner every time."

—Diane Sanfilippo, BS, NC, Certified Nutrition Consultant and author of *Practical Paleo: A Customized Approach to Health and a Whole-Foods Lifestyle*

"Whenever you go on a trip somewhere unfamiliar in your car, you use a GPS to help guide you. But what about an even more important trip through the grocery store, full of all sorts of strange and odd products blaring a multitude of health claims? Couldn't you use a GPS to help point you in the right direction for finding the best possible nutrient-dense foods you can possibly find? If you've been lost and confused, attempting to circumnavigate around your local grocery store, trying to find the best truly healthy foods for your family to eat, then let this book be an eye-opener about exactly what you are putting in your mouth. Trust me, when you find out how much our food supply has been adulterated, you will be left shocked and stunned. After reading Rich Food, Poor Food, you may never eat anything out of a box ever again!"

—Jimmy Moore, Livin' La Vida Low-Carb Blog and Podcast

"Rich Food, Poor Food will take your awareness for healthy food choices to the next level as Jayson and Mira expose the many hidden ingredients in the foods of today. You'll feel as though Jayson and Mira are right there with you as they guide you through the grocery store maze. You will learn how to avoid the snares of misleading health claims and toxic ingredients in our foods, and will emerge from reading this book feeling more confident about how to make better food choices. Whether you are a long-time healthy eater or new to thinking critically about optimal nutritional, there is much to gain in reading Rich Food, Poor Food."

—Hayley Mason and Bill Staley, bestselling authors of *Make it Paleo*

"Finally, a book that tells you what you really need to know to make healthy food choices in the real world. An outstanding addition to any library."

—Jonny Bowden, PhD, CNS, aka "the Rogue Nutritionist," author of *The 150 Healthiest Foods* and *The Great Cholesterol Myth*

"Why has a simple trip to the supermarket become so dangerous? Because the foods you habitually put into your cart now contain more and more questionable ingredients. It's time we all start reading labels properly! Rich Food, Poor Food is the ultimate shopping guide we have all been looking for. You will become informed in this wonderful and practical resource."

—Laurentine ten Bosch, Director and Producer, *Food Matters* and *Hungry For Change*

"After reading through Rich Food, Poor Food, I discovered that a couple of my favorite brands were Poor Foods. When I tried some approved brands to replace my favorites, I discovered they actually tasted better! This book really helps you organize and fine-tune your shopping list to make sure you find the best available products in each category."

—Gail Gilbert
Barview, OR

"The smart grocery buyer has had to learn more and more about the various hidden dangers lurking in innocent-appearing foods, from vegetable oils to fake flavorings to toxins that don't even get disclosed. Yes it's kind of crazy that you now need a book to guide you through the grocery store like it's some kind of foreign country. But rather than curse the darkness, the Caltons cast light. Rich Food, Poor Food is an indispensable source of information that not only succinctly summarizes common points of confusion my patients face when changing their diets, but also is sure to educate even the savviest shopper.

Too few diet books have emphasized anything other than what food manufacturers want us to pay attention to. Rich Food, Poor Food helps us to focus on two things that I find matter most: That foods are grown in healthy soil and then processed in ways that protect or even enhance the nutrient content. This book is colorful and appealing enough, and simple in concept enough, to make a great gift for that person in your life who you think really needs it!"

—Catherine Shanahan, MD. Author of *Deep Nutrition*

"Rich Food, Poor Food is the one new book that every healthy grocery shopper should have in their cart. I recommend to all my clients and athletes when it comes to getting a healthy grocery shopping list and learning exactly how to compare foods at the grocery store. With Rich Food, Poor Food, you're going take an adventure through every aisle of the grocery store and learn the biggest dairy mistakes, whether you can actually find healthy meat at Walmart, how to use the produce numbering system, how to make delicious homemade mayonnaise, what to look for when buying nuts and seeds, how to beat a soda addiction, and much more!"

—Ben Greenfield, Leading low-carb endurance performer, author, speaker, and coach.

"The modern-day supermarket is downright confusing. Rich Food, Poor Food is an essential tool to help us dodge the frankenfoods so we can get straight to the good stuff. Highly recommended!"

—Abel James, author and host of Fat Burning Man podcast show

Introduction

O nce in a blue moon, a book comes along that has the power to start a movement. *Rich Food, Poor Food* is just such a book. You may think that the foods you are buying each week at the grocery store are the "healthiest" options, but what do you really know about BHT, modified cornstarch, partially hydrogenated soybean oil, mono and diglycerides, hydrolyzed corn gluten, autolyzed yeast extract, dextrose, rBGH, or azodicarbonamide—not to mention, GMOs, BPA, BVO, or any of the 150 potentially dangerous and unhealthy Poor Food ingredients the Caltons expose in this must-have grocery store guide? While this stuff clearly sounds unappetizing and unhealthy, the sad truth is that these items are ubiquitous in our friendly neighborhood grocery stores.

Even well-meaning consumers looking to eat as healthy as possible and avoid these crazy chemical additives often fall prey to misleading advertising and marketing gimmicks. In fact, much of what is presented at the grocery stores, convenience stores, and fast-food joints of the Western world is so far removed from its original state that it can scarcely be called food. "Edible food-like substances" is how author Michael Pollan describes the familiar offerings from our favorite food giants.

If you're reading this book, you are likely quite far ahead of the pack when it comes to knowledge and interest about healthy eating. You're likely familiar with the popular adages to avoid foods with stuff you can't pronounce on the label or to shop the perimeter aisles of the grocery store, where the fresh foods are typically located. You may have even embraced the Primal/Paleo/evolutionary health movement and optimized your diet to be free of naked calories and centered upon the micronutrient-rich plant and animal foods that our ancestors evolved on.

One thing's for sure: whoever you are and whatever your current level of knowledge and commitment is, there is always room for improvement. While I've spent years writing and researching about health and nutrition, I have learned a great deal from my association with the Caltons and their focus on maximizing micronutrient values (vitamins, minerals, antioxidants, essential amino and fatty acids) and avoiding potentially harmful ingredients. And while there are great many books, websites, and diet gurus out there today dispensing sound (and unsound!) nutritional advice, *Rich Food, Poor Food* is one of the best books I have ever read, taking the idea of food quality to a completely new level and offering quick and easy recipes, money-saving tips, and even exclusive Rich Food coupons just for you. It is a simple, straightforward, logical approach to smart grocery shopping that has the ability to change your life, and forever change the way you shop for food.

Whether you're deep into healthful eating or just grabbed this book to pick up a few shopping tips to help your family, you'll find the material easy to understand, fun to learn, and extremely valuable to your health and well-being. You will no longer be a victim of manipulative marketing messages that entice you to consume something presented as "healthy," "lean," "natural," or the like in the name of health. Each time you visit the grocery store, you'll feel confident and empowered that you are taking control of your health. Instead of succumbing to the blizzard of signs, specials, coupons, and campaigns, you'll feel like the guy or gal with an authentic treasure map, effortlessly navigating the crowded aisles, knowing exactly what you are looking for. You'll expand your shopping scope beyond trudging to the closest supermarket chain, and instead learn how to tap into the ultimate potential of your community to deliver the healthiest and most enjoyable snacks and meals to your home!

By the time you are finished with *Rich Food, Poor Food,* you will have all the knowledge you need to make smart and safe decisions concerning the food you are purchasing for your family. And for all you Primal, Paleo, and wheat-sensitive eaters out there—each and every recommended Rich Food is wheat free. *Rich Food, Poor Food* is the *Eat This, Not That* for health-conscious individuals. Buy it, read it, and join the Rich Food Revolution!

In Good Health,

Mark Sisson
Malibu, CA
January 2013

PART ONE

Know Before You Go

Chapter One

Your Rich Food Road Trip

I magine your next visit to the grocery store as an adventurous road trip, on which instead of visiting museums or the largest ball of twine, or navigating highways and back roads, your shopping expedition takes place up and down numerous aisles filled with thousands of products. The mission: to find the freshest, healthiest choices for the foods on your shopping list.

You will pass tempting billboards willing you to go off course in the form of advertisements, sale signs, misleading packaging, and in-aisle displays. The images and slogans on the boxes, bags, and brightly colored bottles pop off the shelves in an attempt to entice you to impulsively add them to your grocery cart. The cartoon characters, strategically placed in a child's line of site, lower on the shelves, call to impressionable children. Claims of heart health, high omega-3s, low calories, low sodium, diet, and all-natural bait you and cause confusion when trying to determine the most nutritious foods.

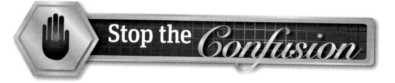

Now imagine this same trip to the grocery store using the *Rich Food, Poor Food* GPS (Grocery Purchasing System). We have programmed this GPS to successfully navigate you through the nutritional chaos, guiding you directly to the healthiest, most micronutrient Rich Foods and re-routing you when you run into dangerous, unhealthy Poor Food choices (sometimes taking you somewhere other than your usual grocery store to find Rich Food choices). By using your *Rich Food, Poor Food* GPS, you will no longer be overwhelmed in the grocery store when trying to choose the healthiest options in each aisle or wonder what makes one brand better for you than another. As your GPS guides you through the nearly forty thousand items populating the average supermarket today, it will give you important nutritional information and interesting food facts and teach you how to decipher the often extensive and intimidating lists of ingredients on food packages. Your new knowledge will help you identify which ingredients are dangerous and unhealthy *before* you purchase them.

The Invention of the Rich Food,
Poor Food Grocery Purchasing System

IN OUR FIRST BOOK, *Naked Calories,* we introduced the incredible discovery we made during the Calton Project, our six-year, one hundred–country research expedition in which we studied the dietary and lifestyle habits of remote, semi-remote, and urban peoples around the world. Based on our observations of these different cultures, which include remote groups deep inside the Amazon, rarely visited tribes of Papua New Guinea, and the bustling urban cities of India and China, we were able to make several unique conclusions about the causation of health and disease.

The first and perhaps most important conclusion was that *micronutrient deficiency* is the most widespread and dangerous health condition of the twenty-first century. Micronutrient deficiency is a state in which our bodies do not obtain the minimum daily requirements of essential vitamins, minerals, and fatty acids. Our research proved that due to soil depletion, global food distribution, factory farming, and modern cooking and food processing methods, the world is in the midst of a micronutrient deficiency pandemic. The danger comes from the fact that modern science now points to these same micronutrient deficiencies as contributing factors in many of today's most prevalent health conditions and chronic diseases.

Reversing Mira's advanced osteoporosis by making her once micronutrient-depleted body sufficient in these health-promoting factors inspired our mission to share with the world our realistic and sustainable program for achieving optimal health.

The first part of that mission was achieved when we published *Naked Calories*, which outlined our three-step approach to micronutrient sufficiency and introduced our Rich Food, Poor Food philosophy. The Rich Food, Poor Food philosophy states that regardless of which diet profile one follows (low-fat, low-carb, Primal/paleo, low-calorie, vegan, vegetarian, etc.), the ultimate goal should be to reach a micronutrient-sufficient state. Consuming as many micronutrient-Rich Foods as possible helps achieve optimal health—preventing disease while naturally increasing youthful energy.

While *Naked Calories* introduced our Rich Food, Poor Food philosophy, many readers suggested that we write a companion food guide to help micronutrient-sufficiency seekers identify Rich Foods as they navigate the supermarket. So, we created this Grocery Purchasing System (GPS) to help identify Rich Foods and avoid Poor Foods in each and every aisle.

In *Rich Food, Poor Food*, we take your food and nutrition knowledge to next level. No longer will the only villains in your foods be Everyday Micronutrient Depleters (EMDs), those stealth thieves we introduced you to in *Naked Calories* that rob you of your essential vitamins, minerals and fatty acids. This indispensable grocery store guide raises the bar on food quality as it teaches you how to quickly identify dangerous food additives, GMOs, and potentially problematic and sinister ingredients.

RICH FOODS = natural, unprocessed, or minimally processed foods that are high in micronutrient content to help you increase your micronutrient-sufficiency levels and are low or void of problematic ingredients that can put your health at risk.

POOR FOODS = highly processed foods that are low or devoid of micronutrients, decreasing your micronutrient sufficiency level, and often contain sinister EMDs alongside numerous other problematic ingredients.

We've read the labels, weighed the information, and programmed your Grocery Purchasing System with the locations of our go-to Rich Food choices. Along your journey, the GPS shares money-saving tips, homemade options, methods on how to lock in a food's nutritional value during preservation and preparation, and much more. Regardless of your age, dietary preference, or current health, *Rich Food, Poor Food* turns your grocery store into your micronutrient pharmacy, filling your shopping cart with a natural prescription for better health and longevity.

Don't worry—we're not going to suggest flavorless, difficult-to-find foods or expensive specialty items or recommend a boring culinary lifestyle. Quite the contrary! This guide is packed with our Rich Food brand-name picks for snacks, sauces, hot dogs, desserts, and other fun foods.

How Is the Rich Food, Poor Food GPS Different?

IN CASE YOU'RE WONDERING if *Rich Food, Poor Food* is just like those other "food swap" guides, it's not. Nowhere in these pages will we tell you to choose Hostess Twinkies over Ding Dongs like those other guys do. (Breaking News: Hostess announces bankruptcy in late 2012 . . . good riddance!) We aren't going to grade the foods on their calorie, sodium, and fat content alone. We feel we would be doing you a disservice by telling you that there is anything even remotely good in either a Twinkie or a Ding Dong! Their top pick, Twinkies, contains thirty-nine ingredients. That's far too many to be considered a Rich Food option. To add insult to injury, high fructose corn syrup, refined white flour, and trans fats make the top five ingredients. We don't very much care that they are only 150 calories each or that they deliver a mere 4.5 grams of fat. The important question, in our opinion, is: Do they deliver health? To answer this, we would ask ourselves, *Is this "food-like substance" the best snack choice, offering high-micronutrient content with few suspect ingredients?* It most certainly is not. And, even if it were, eating low-fat, low-calorie, micronutrient-deficient Twinkies does not necessarily aid in weight loss or weight maintenance. In fact, in *Naked Calories,* we illustrated how eating a micronutrient-sufficient diet, even if it is considered a higher-fat or higher-calorie food choice, can contribute to greater weight loss and health benefits than eating a micronutrient-deficient, low-calorie, low-fat "food-like" substance.

For the sake of cutting calories and fat, food quality has been ignored, and we are paying the price for this with our health. This GPS guide, unlike others before it, values food quality above all else. What determines food quality? Well, food quality is based on two factors: what food delivers to your body and what it leaves out.

First, is the food rich in micronutrients? Meaning, does the food deliver the best-quality, natural ingredients, and is it highest in the essential vitamins, minerals, and fatty acids required daily to obtain and sustain optimal health? Second, your GPS ensures that Poor Food ingredients that can rob you of your essential micronutrients and be detrimental to your health do not sneak into your cart and end up on your plate. To put it plainly, your GPS directs you to Rich Food choices that put the good things in and leave bad things out.

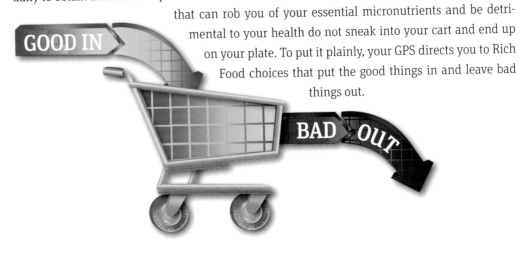

· · · · · · · · · · · · · · · ·

Deciphering the Modern Food Package

THIS IS WHERE IT ALL BEGINS. As we stated earlier, it is inevitable that you will be bombarded with billboards in the form of food packages and advertisements during your grocery store road trip. Let's face it, modern food packages are an advertising masterpiece. In the very best of cases, they educate you as to the true wholesome goodness of a product. In the very worst of cases, they are designed to deceive you with a flashy promise on the front of the package, distracting your attention from the unhealthy truths hidden on the back of the package on the rarely read ingredient list. As has often been said about the used car market, the supermarket has truly become a "buyer beware" environment. Due to this unfortunate reality, we want to give you the lay of the label, so to speak. A quick lesson in "supermarket smarts" will help you successfully identify foods that are delivering healthy nutrition and steer clear of those foods designed to *sound healthy that are really only deceiving you with advertising jargon.*

The Lay of the Label—Beware of the Con Artist

TRUE STORY: We once bought a used vehicle from a man named Cia Kahn (pronounced *See A Con*). Get it? Not an ideal name for a used car salesman, and one that made us investigate his claims with a fine-tooth comb. Luckily for us, the vehicle we purchased turned out to be everything good old Cia Kahn said it was and more. However, most of the brand names in the grocery store don't conjure up the images of dishonesty like Cia Kahn's name did, begging you to investigate them further. Instead, brand names like Quaker, Healthy Choice, Pepperidge Farms, and Gerber bring to mind things like strong moral character, health, and wholesomeness. Their good names are meant to lull you into a false sense of security. But don't be fooled by these slick corporate identifiers and think that you don't need to investigate their products. By learning the lay of the label, you will easily be able to "see a con" from a mile away! So, let's get started.

Divide and Conquer

The strategic genius of the divide-and-conquer philosophy has stood the test of time, and that is why we are going to use it to conquer today's food package. By understanding each section of your food's packaging, you will be able to masterfully discern whether you are about to buy a Rich Food or a Poor Food. Let's start by dividing the packaged food into three basic parts:

1. The front, or "billboard"
2. The Nutrition Facts, often referred to as "the label"
3. The all-important, but often overlooked, ingredient list

Most of us are more than familiar with the front of the food package. Some of us may read a label now and again. But most of us rarely, if ever, spend time reading ingredient lists. As you will discover, however, the ingredient list is the last bastion of hope for health-conscious consumers trying to uncover the true facts about what is in their food.

To illustrate just how misleading packaging can be, let's use our divide-and-conquer technique to compare two products manufactured by the same company.

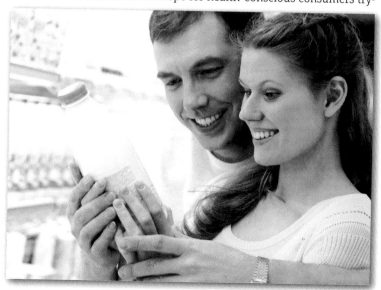

Lay's Classic Potato Chips vs. Baked! Lay's Original Potato Crisps

LET'S BEGIN THIS COMPARISON by examining these products exactly the same way the manufacturers design them to be seen: face-first. Whether a box, bag, bottle, tub, or can, the first step is to consider the front of the package for what it really is—a billboard. Take a moment to look at the two images of Lay's potato chips to the right. What difference do you notice first? What is their marketing team trying to convince you of? The most dramatic difference is in the look and texture of the two bags. The Classic Potato Chips are in a shiny bag with bright colors, whereas the baked chips are in a softly textured bag with warmer, muted colors designed to make them look more natural so you feel better about buying them.

The next change was made to the Lay's logo, which, as you can see, was shrunk considerably for the baked version and replaced with a new headline—a huge "Baked!" spanning the width of the bag. This is their way of saying—no, *screaming*—"Healthy!" or "Not fried!" Additionally, an official-looking seal has been added, touting healthy claims to further imply a healthy message. It appears as though this baked product, unlike the classic Lay's, is now all-natural, with no MSG, no preservatives, and no artificial flavors.

Finally, did you notice that one product is called "chips," while the other is called "crisps?" At first, we didn't. The graphic designers purposefully placed this barely legible identifier at the bottom left-hand corner of the bag. Sometimes it is the details that are buried in the billboard's flash that become the most important clues.

Forget about whether you like baked crisps or potato chips at all. Just ask yourself these questions: How do you feel when you look at each bag, and what is the message that Lay's has spent millions of dollars to convey? If you answered that the Baked! Lay's Original Potato Crisps are a healthier, smarter snack, you're right! But are you really right? Is the baked crisp really healthier? Are they really a smarter choice than the old, fried version of the Lay's Classic? Let's continue our head-to-head comparison by next looking at the label, or Nutrition Facts, on both bags to see what information we gather there.

As you turn the bag around, the cold, hard facts stare you in the face: calories, fat, carbohydrate, protein, and numerous micronutrient levels in our foods are revealed. This is where the other "swap" books tell you to focus your attention. *Eat This, Not That,* for instance, alludes to the idea that everything you need to know in order to make a logical, and seemingly valid, argument in favor of the Baked! Lay's as a better choice than the classic fried version is found here.

The Baked! Lay's total calories have gone from 160 to 120 per serving. That is a 25 percent reduction.

 CHECK ONE.

Sodium has gone from 170 mg to 135 mg—a 21 percent reduction.

 CHECK TWO.

Fat has an enormous reduction of 80 percent—10 grams to 2 grams.

 CHECK THREE.

Even the 1.5 grams of saturated fat in the fried chips has been reduced by 100 percent to 0 grams in the crisps. Yes, sir, you don't have to be a rocket scientist to see that the baked crisps check all the boxes for healthy, smarter snacking—if what we consider healthy is only lower calories, lower sodium, and lower fat.

But don't be sold after inspecting only this portion of the information. There are other numbers in the Nutrition Facts that *Eat This, Not That* doesn't encourage readers to consider. Did you notice that the carbohydrates increased from 15 to 23 grams per serving? Or that the sugar more than doubled? That seems odd, doesn't it? Why didn't they bring that to our attention? For the more than 100 million Americans who are diabetic or pre-diabetic, knowing the sugar content is important! Our point here is that the Nutrition Facts can only tell you one thing: whether the fats, carbohydrates, sugars, and protein levels fit in to your dietary profile. That's it, folks. It reports the numbers—and nothing more.

If you are a low-fat dieter, you can scan the Nutrition Facts for low-fat indicators; alternatively, low-carb dieters can search labels for low-carbohydrate values. While it is still important to read the Nutrition Facts to determine whether a food follows your dietary guidelines, it cannot help you determine if it is a Rich Food or Poor Food.

Nutrition Facts
Serving Size 1 oz. (28g/About 15 chips)

Amount Per Serving

Calories 160	Calories from Fat 90
	% Daily Value*
Total Fat 10g	**16%**
Saturated Fat 1.5g	**8%**
Trans Fat 0g	
Cholesterol 0mg	**0%**
Sodium 170mg	**7%**
Potassium 350mg	**10%**
Total Carbohydrate 15g	**5%**
Dietary Fiber 1g	**5%**
Sugars less than 1g	
Protein 2g	

Vitamin A 0%	•	Vitamin C 10%
Calcium 0%	•	Iron 2%
Vitamin E 6%	•	Thiamin 4%
Niacin 6%	•	Vitamin B6 10%
Magnesium 4%	•	Zinc 2%

Nutrition Facts
Serving Size 1 oz. (28g/About 15 crisps)

Amount Per Serving

Calories 120	Calories from Fat 20
	% Daily Value*
Total Fat 2g	**3%**
Saturated Fat 0g	**0%**
Trans Fat 0g	
Cholesterol 0mg	**0%**
Sodium 135mg	**6%**
Potassium 270mg	**8%**
Total Carbohydrate 23g	**8%**
Dietary Fiber 2g	**7%**
Sugars 2g	
Protein 2g	

Vitamin A 0%	•	Vitamin C 4%
Calcium 0%	•	Iron 2%
Thiamin 6%	•	Riboflavin 2%
Niacin 6%	•	Vitamin B6 15%
Phosphorus 4%	•	Magnesium 4%

MIRA USED TO FOLLOW A LOW-FAT DIET. She was programmed to pick up a food, read the nutrition facts, and choose only the foods that were less than 100 calories with no more than 1 gram of fat per serving. To her, that was smart and healthy, because she was told that choosing foods by reading the label was what smart and healthy people do. What she learned was that many of her "smart" foods were full of Naked Calories and were micronutrient-deficient Poor Foods, which eventually led her to develop advanced osteoporosis at thirty years of age! Oh, she was thin, all right, but far from healthy.

We are not saying that just because a food is 100 calories or less and 1 gram of fat or less means it is bad for you—there are low-fat Rich Foods and low-fat Poor Foods; low-carbohydrate Rich Foods and low-carbohydrate Poor Foods. We're saying, take a moment to take the next step and investigate the ingredient list before you assume it's a smart and healthy choice—because *that's what smart and healthy people do.*

The Road Less Traveled

So off we go to inspect the ingredient list—the spot where the rubber hits the road. If you had listened to *Eat This, Not That,* you might never set foot in this direction, even though this is the most important part of the product's package.

Take a moment to look at the ingredients in the Lay's Classic chips. They have only three ingredients: potatoes, vegetable oil,

> **Ingredients:** Potatoes, Vegetable Oil (Sunflower, Corn and/or Canola Oil), and Salt.

and salt. Granted, they are not organic potatoes, organic palm oil, or unrefined salt, which we'd prefer, but on the whole, there are no EMDs, carcinogens, toxic additives, or unpronounceable names. The general rule of thumb, remember, is that the fewer the ingredients, the better food, so this is a wee bit confusing, as the last we checked, three is a pretty low number where ingredients are concerned.

Now, let's look at the healthier, smarter baked potato chips—oops, we mean *crisps*. Wow! Really? We expected the Baked! Lay's potato crisps to be baked slices of potato with less oil and a little less salt—in essence, a lower-fat (healthier and smarter) version of the classic Lay's potato chip. Boy, did we have egg on our faces. While Lay's may have started with good intentions, somewhere, they took a very wrong turn.

Just look at the list of ingredients that make up this "Franken Chip" lab experiment. Dried potatoes (what—like potato flakes or granules?), cornstarch (oh, so now

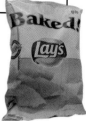

Ingredients: Dried Potatoes, Cornstarch, Sugar, Corn Oil, Salt, Soy Lecithin, and Corn Sugar. **CONTAINS A SOY INGREDIENT.**

these are corn crisps, too?), sugar (precisely what a healthier, smarter snack should not include), corn oil (this has Genetically Modified Organism—GMO—written all over it), salt (not unrefined salt), soy lecithin (and it's a soy chip, too—GMO alert!), and corn sugar (aka high fructose corn syrup). We'll cover these Poor Food ingredients in the next chapter.

This is no joke. This is the real ingredient list on the baked crisps. This lower-calorie, low-fat snack is *not* a healthier, smarter choice. It is very definitely a Poor Food choice with ingredients that may be linked to cancer, diabetes, high blood pressure, obesity, infertility, compromised immunity, accelerated aging, and numerous other health conditions and diseases. Had you purchased this product only after a review of the Nutrition Facts, you would have opened yourself up to unwanted ingredients.

When Eat This, Not That named these potato crisps their go-to chip choice, they boasted, "Baked! Lay's represents the classic potato chip at its absolute best." What? Are they serious? These crisps are not even made with real potato slices. Far from the absolute best, the Baked! Lay's represents to us just how far we have strayed from natural foods and onto a dangerous new path paved with highly processed, manufactured food-like substances.

You can now see that it is only by reading the ingredient list that you can easily differentiate a Rich Food from a Poor Food, even when both the billboard and Nutrition Facts may be trying to deceive you. And while this comparison contest hopefully enlightened you to the nature of misleading packaging, let us also point out that the winner of this battle has no cause for celebration. Any way you slice them (literally), Lay's potato chips are a Poor Food; they're empty calories, with infinitesimal micronutrients and numerous health-compromising ingredients. To locate a true Rich Food chip, visit Aisle 8: Snacks.

The Rich Food, Poor Food GPS guides you to the Rich Food choices available in every aisle. We have identified the products with ingredients that support health. On those occasions, however, when the brand we suggest is not available, or you don't find one of your favorite foods listed in this book, you will have the tools to help you divide and conquer the packaging on your own to determine the best brand for you.

But wait. It is a dangerous world out there. In order to succeed in the stores, you'll need a quick lesson in GPS Operations.

THE OWNER'S MANUAL

Now that you know how we identify Rich Foods and divide and conquer food packaging, it is time you become acquainted with the recurring features that will assist you in your shopping experience.

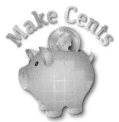

Choosing quality foods can cost a little more because they contain wholesome, expensive ingredients in lieu of cheap, health-depleting ones. But this GPS not only rewards your health, it rewards your checkbook, too. Our Make Cents tips offer cash-conserving suggestions that will help you lower the tolls on your highway to health.

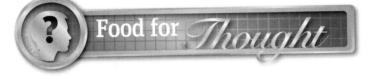

These fun facts really give you something to think about and help bring to life the truth about the safety, nutrition, and nature of food products. Here, your GPS supplies you with some of the fine print that may give you pause the next time you peruse the aisles. Curious about coffee? Wondering about wheat? Food for Thought is information for the most inquisitive of minds.

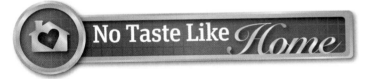

Micronutrient depleters, toxic carcinogens, and sugar substitutes—oh, my! Sometimes the road to finding a Rich Food is fraught with health-violating villains. When this happens, your GPS saves the day and sends you home with a do-it-yourself, homemade solution.

STEER HERE Want to know which hot dog is a hero? Are you searching for the perfect pasta sauce? No matter which aisle you are shopping in, we have identified our go-to Rich Food choices that put the good things in and leave the bad things out. Put the pedal to the metal and get in the fast lane because it couldn't get any easier than this. This GPS is programmed to direct you to hundreds of our fantastic Rich Food choices that have won our seal of approval. We've named names and programmed the GPS with the products that satisfy our Rich Food rules.

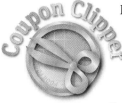

In our Steer Here section, you will find our coupon clipper icons next to some of our Rich Food options. When you see the symbol next to a product's name, there is a money-saving coupon waiting for you in our Rich Food Resource Center on our website, CaltonNutrition.com. Skip the Sunday papers—manufacturers usually only offer savings on their highly processed foods. Our collection of online coupons makes Rich Foods more affordable—trimming the costs without trimming the quality.

STEER CLEAR

Put your hands behind your back, and step away from the shopping cart! The foods that make this list are in serious violation of the Rich Food rules. If we were the food police, we would give out major fines to these offenders. They may contain Everyday Micronutrient Depleters (EMDs), food thickeners, artificial colors, or other Poor Food ingredients outlined in the next chapter. However, this "do not buy" list is far from complete. In fact, many other similar pothole products exist. This GPS feature is set to remind you of common problems in this food category, allowing you to become fluent in Poor Food labeling lingo and steer clear of nutrition violators.

We are not attacking manufacturers, nor are we telling you to boycott their products. You will see in these Steer Clear sections that we are pinpointing Poor Food ingredients in products that we consider to be poor choices for reaching micronutrient sufficiency. We would love for manufacturers who make our lists to take these suggestions to heart. You never know—with a few recipe altera- tions, these products might someday go from Steer Clear to Steer Here.

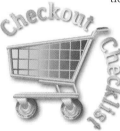

You may be thinking, *How does this GPS even know what grocery store I shop at or which products they sell?* You got us . . . it doesn't. In fact, we can't guarantee which Steer Here products will be available in your market. However, we have designed a solution called the Checkout Checklist.

If you find that our Steer Here Rich Food choices are not sold in your store, head directly to the Checkout Checklist, where we outline what good things to look for in the product you are considering and what bad things to avoid. The checklist reminds you of what made our Steer Here products so appealing to us and warns you of Poor Food ingredients. Regardless of where you are shopping, following the Checkout Checklist will make for a successful grocery shopping experience. Make sure to write down the name of the product you have selected in the spaces provided to save you time and energy the next time you hit the aisles.

Even with nearly forty thousand items to choose from, sometimes the supermarket is woefully deficient in Rich Food options. On these occasions, we will find you an alternate route to health and direct you out of the grocery store to a new location where the Richest Foods can be found. Maybe it is a little extra work or a few extra miles out of your way. Perhaps, at first glance, it may even cost you a bit more. However, we are confident that you will soon recognize that the superiority of these selections is worth every ounce of extra effort. The savvy shopper knows that taking alternate routes every once in a while can save you precious time and money in the long run.

RICH FOOD vs POOR FOOD

If you read *Naked Calories,* you may remember these head-to-head analyses of two seemingly similar products. We stack up our Rich Food choice next to a Poor Food option to show you just how far superior they really are. Higher in micronutrients? Lower in added sugars? When you encounter these diagrams, you will have a clear picture as to just how important making these food swaps can be to your health.

Now that you know how to use this book, let's shift gears and get acquainted with the cast of unsavory characters you will encounter along your Rich Food shopping excursion. Meeting this cast will help you demystify many of the terms you will see on the ingredient list. This next chapter will serve as an important reference guide for all the aisles to come because these label losers keep popping up everywhere.

Chapter 2
Problematic Personalities

We are about to introduce you to a pack of problematic personalities you will encounter during your grocery store expedition. Don't let these numerous names overwhelm you—your GPS operating system is already programmed to steer clear of these Poor Food perpetrators. Keep this guide handy when you shop to reference an ingredient's rap sheet whenever you are in doubt.

Everyday Micronutrient Depleters (EMDs)

IN *NAKED CALORIES,* we introduced you to a myriad of micronutrient thieves called Everyday Micronutrient Depleters (EMDs). While we went into each of the five EMDs in detail in *Naked Calories,* here is a quick review. By avoiding these EMDs, you can increase the amount of health-enhancing micronutrients that your food delivers with every delicious bite.

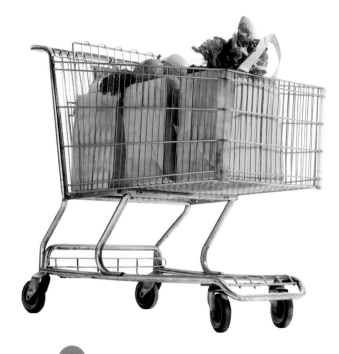

Travel Time and Storage

EMD 1

EXPRESS LANE MESSAGE: The longer or farther your food travels to your table, the fewer micronutrients it will deliver. This holds true for all fresh foods—from carrots to chicken, apples to spinach.

YOUR GPS DIRECTS YOU TO: Locally grown and raised foods. Local and organic is even better.

Unnatural Feed and Environment

EMD 2

EXPRESS LANE MESSAGE: Animals living in overcrowded factory farm conditions and given feed that is unnatural to their species are less nutritious than those raised on smaller, family-run farms and fed their natural diet.

YOUR GPS DIRECTS YOU TO: Grass-fed beef and dairy products, wild-caught fish, pastured chickens and eggs.

Pasteurization

EMD 3

EXPRESS LANE MESSAGE: Pasteurizing dairy products reduces their micronutrient content and denatures their proteins (more on this in the Dairy section). Cold pasteurization, known as irradiation, which typically affects produce, spices, and meats, also diminishes vitamins and minerals while creating dangerous, health-hindering "free radicals" (atoms, molecules, or ions that contain unpaired electrons and crash into each other, multiplying exponentially) that contribute to many degenerative diseases, including heart disease, dementia, cancer, and cataracts.

YOUR GPS DIRECTS YOU TO: Unpasteurized (raw) dairy and organic foods. Note: Seeing *organic* on a label ensures a product has not been irradiated but does not ensure dairy or other products have not been pasteurized.

Freezing and Canning

EMD 4

EXPRESS LANE MESSAGE: Fresh is only more micro-nutrient dense than frozen or canned if it is *very* fresh (local or regional).

YOUR GPS DIRECTS YOU TO IN ORDER OF PREFERENCE: Fresh and local, those picked at peak of ripeness for flash-freezing or canning (in BPA-free cans).

Peeling and Cooking Methods

EXPRESS LANE MESSAGE:

EMD 5

Leave the skin on organic or well-washed vegetables to maximize micronutrients. Leave foods whole (uncut) until just before serving to reduce oxidation and micronutrient loss. Cook foods minimally and, when possible, avoid reheating meals to prevent a reduction in their vitamin and mineral levels.

YOUR GPS DIRECTS YOU TO: Fresh, uncut, uncooked foods. Avoid premade, microwavable, and even grocery store–prepared items.

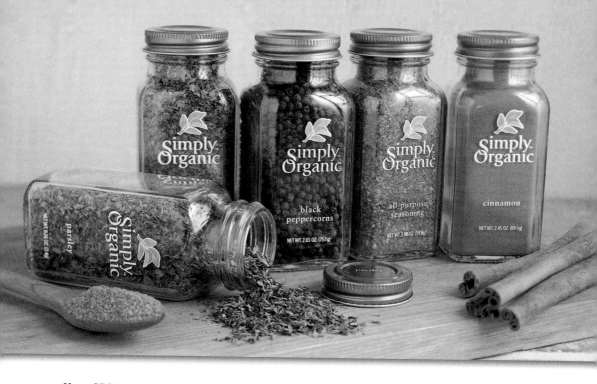

Your GPS is programmed to direct you to foods that avoid the aforementioned five Everyday Micronutrient Depleters. So, for example, a hot dog made from organic, grass-fed beef and organic spices will rate higher, or will be considered a Richer Food, than a regular beef hot dog with regular spices—even if the regular hot dog is lower in calories, sodium, and fat. That just makes sense, doesn't it? A hot dog made from factory-farmed beef, fed an unnatural, corn-based diet, shot up with antibiotics and hormones, and flavored with irradiated, free radical-filled spices is never going to be as healthy as one made from humanely raised, organic, grass-fed beef, free of hormones and antibiotics, prepared with organic spices without free radicals.

It all comes down to food quality and understanding that choosing foods that are made using high-quality, wholesome, micronutrient-rich ingredients is nature's prescription to optimal health. While that factory-farmed, micronutrient-deficient frank may deliver the antiquated and faulty prescription for health (low-calorie, low-sodium, and low-fat), it does not deliver nature's prescription.

Above and beyond directing you to the products that increase micronutrient content by upping food quality, your GPS avoids additional EMDs. These infamous micronutrient-depleting ingredients are found in a disturbing variety of foods and drinks. They are even found in some foods and drinks labeled "healthy" and "natural." Some of them are added into products, while others are naturally occurring—but either way, they need to be recognized for their micronutrient-robbing effects. Sometimes, these EMDs are found in nutritious fruits and vegetables. It is not our goal to have you remove all of these from your diet, but rather to understand their micronutrient-depleting effects so that you can have a clearer picture of your micronutrient sufficiency level.

Criminal EMDs	Guilty of	Usual Hangouts & Aliases
SUGAR	Depleting vitamin C due to competition for cell entry. Being stripped and refined of all of its own micronutrients; upsetting the mineral relationships in the body. Causing chromium and copper deficiencies. Blocking the absorption of calcium and magnesium. Being more addictive than cocaine (as discussed in *Naked Calories*). Spiking insulin due to it raising blood sugar. Table sugar measures a 60 on the glycemic index. The glycemic index tell us which foods raise glucose levels fastest and highest on a scale of 0 to 100. Foods with a glycemic load over 55 are considered high. Eating too many foods with high glycemic index levels can lead to insulin resistance and diabetes.	**FOUND IN:** Sodas, dessert items, candies, frozen fruits and vegetables, sauces, soups, and the vast majority of products in the supermarket. GMO ALERT! Fifty-five percent of all sugar in processed foods is from genetically modified beets—see page 27 for details. **ALIASES INCLUDE:** Agave nectar, brown sugar, cane crystals, cane sugar, caramel, crystalline fructose, dextrose, evaporated cane juice, fructose, fruit juice concentrate, glucose, honey, invert sugar, lactose, maltose, malt syrup, molasses, raw sugar, sucrose, and syrup.
HIGH FRUCTOSE CORN SYRUP (HFCS)	Soil erosion causing fewer micronutrients in our foods. Depleting chromium, magnesium, zinc, and copper from the body. Not triggering leptin, which causes overeating. Causing insulin spike due to its high glycemic index of 73.	**FOUND IN:** Nearly every aisle in the grocery store. The USDA reports that the average American consumes 63 pounds of HFCS a year. Twenty percent of all calories children consume are from HFCS. **ALIASES INCLUDE:** Corn sweetener, corn syrup , corn sugar.
PHYTIC ACID (PHYTATES)	Blocking the absorption of calcium, magnesium, copper, manganese, chromium, iron, zinc, and niacin. Accelerating the metabolism of vitamin D, thus using your reserves faster.	**FOUND IN:** Numerous healthy fruits and vegetables, in acceptable amounts, but in excess in nuts, seeds, and grains, especially whole grains (wheat, rice, pasta, corn, cereal, cooking grains).

Criminal EMDs	Guilty of	Usual Hangouts & Aliases
OXALIC ACID (OXALATES)	Binding to calcium, magnesium, and iron, which blocks their absorption.	FOUND IN: Chocolate, seeds, nuts, spinach, beans, collard greens, potatoes, artichokes, squash, wheat bran, quinoa, beets, and soy products.
CAFFEINE	Slightly reducing calcium levels.	FOUND IN: Coffees and teas, chocolate, hot cocoa, chocolate ice creams, and energy drinks.
ALCOHOL	Inhibiting the breakdown of micro-nutrients by decreasing digestive enzyme secretion when consumed in excess. Damaging the cells that line the stomach and intestines and disabling transport of some micronutrients into the blood.	FOUND IN: Wine, wine coolers, beer, champagne, hard liquor, hard cider, and grain alcohol.
PHOSPHORIC ACID	Increasing the excretion of calcium and impairing the absorption of both calcium and magnesium.	FOUND IN: Soda, flavored waters, and some foods.
TANNINS	Negatively influences iron and calcium absorption. Some studies indicate magnesium and zinc absorption may also be affected.	FOUND IN: Red wine, berries, tea, fruit juices, spices, and nuts.

The EMD Rap Sheet

Now that you are aware of these stealth little thieves called EMDs that are lurking in your foods and beverages, it's time we introduce you to a second slew of detrimental deviants usually found hanging out in the general vicinity of the EMDs. Birds of a feather flock together, so when you see one of the following ingredients on a label, you are likely to find others hiding in there as well.

Sinister Sugar Substitutes

MEET THE SINISTER SUGAR SUBSTI-
TUTES (SSS). Unlike the EMDs sugar and high
fructose corn syrup, the SSS don't rob you of
your micronutrients. However, scientific data
suggests that they can be just as detrimental
to your health. Let's get acquainted with these
sweet suspects and find out how they may be
blocking your road to optimal health.

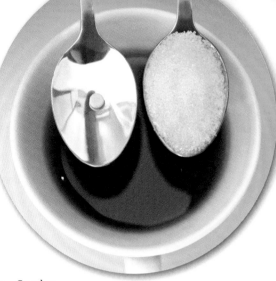

Sucralose

KNOWN ALIASES: Splenda, Sukrana, SucraPlus, Candys,
Cukren, Nevella, and E955 (European Union).

RECENT SIGHTINGS: Pepsi ONE, Breyers CarbSmart ice cream, Maple Grove Farms sugar-free
syrup, Diet Rite cola, Propel water, Diet V8 Splash.

SUSPECTED OF: According to a Duke University study, sucralose decreased "good" gut bacteria by
50 percent. Your gut is home to 80 percent of your immune system, and these same bacteria can
help fight heart disease, reduce cravings, and, best of all, aid in the absorption of your micronutrients. While it is the least criminal of the sugar substitute squad and deemed safe by the Center
for Science in the Public Interest, avoid sucralose whenever possible.

Acesulfame Potassium

KNOWN ALIASES: Acesulfame K, Sunett, Sweet One, and E950 (European Union).

RECENT SIGHTINGS: Diet Rite cola, Pepsi Max, Coca-Cola Zero, Fresca, Wrigley's spearmint gum,
some SoBe products, and Sugar-Free Jell-O.

SUSPECTED OF: This sweetener rarely works a job alone. You can frequently find it as an ingredient alongside sucralose or aspartame. It is known to increase insulin release and has been linked
to thyroid tumors.

Aspartame

KNOWN ALIASES: NutraSweet, Equal, AminoSweet, Canderel, Spoonful, Equal-Measure, and
E951 (European Union).

RECENT SIGHTINGS: Diet Coke, 7up Free, Ocean Spray On the Go, Yoplait Light, Wrigley's Orbit
gum (all varieties), and more than six thousand other grocery store products.

SUSPECTED OF: Aspartame accounts for more than 75 percent of all adverse reactions to food
additives reported to the FDA and has been well reported to cause neurological symptoms

like dizziness, seizures, depression, breathing difficulties, and weight gain. Some studies have even linked it to cancer, epilepsy, Alzheimer's, and multiple sclerosis. Aspartame contains methanol, which converts to formaldehyde—that's right, the same stuff used to embalm a corpse. This offender should be avoided at all costs.

GUILTY OF: Spiking insulin and leptin levels! Remember that insulin is our fat storage hormone. This means that while you may choose this sweetener to lose weight, you may actually pack on the pounds. In *Naked Calories,* we learned that leptin is the hormone that tells your body you are full. Overstimulation of leptin makes your body "deaf" to its message that you are full, which is a dieter's disaster because your body learns to ignore satiation.

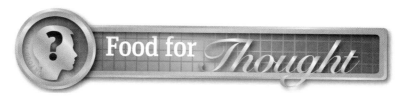

Recent studies have proven that choosing foods and beverages sweetened with sugar substitutes may actually cause you to overeat and gain weight and slow down your metabolism. While these Sinister Sugar Substitutes may lull you in to a false sense of zero-calorie security, your body is less convinced. The sweetness tells your brain that calories and micronutrients are coming in; however, when they don't arrive, your body shouts out for nutrients and sends you on a quest to find more food.

Neotame

KNOWN ALIASES: Aspartame with a neo (new) name and a worse attitude. Also known as E961 (European Union).

RECENT SIGHTINGS: Ultimate Nutrition Protein Isolate chocolate cream shake, SunnyD Tangy Original punch, Weight Watchers cherry cheesecake nonfat yogurt, Detour protein bars, Hostess 100-Calorie Packs.

SUSPECTED OF: A new-and-improved version of the SSS aspartame, neotame is the fastest growing sweetener on the market. Why? It's been updated to be sweeter, and it no longer requires specialized warnings on the label. You may wonder how its creator Monsanto altered the potentially neurologically harmful aspartame to make it safe. Well, neotame still contains all the dangerous elements found in aspartame, but it has one added ingredient called 3,3-dimethylbutyraldehyde that makes it safer for those suffering from certain rare health conditions (such as phenylketonuria, or PKU for short) to consume.

Because it is now safer for this small group of individuals, the government no longer requires this new version of aspartame to be specially labeled. But what is 3,3-dimethylbutyraldehyde?

Believe it or not, your food has been made "safer" by adding an ingredient that is labeled as a highly flammable irritant to skin, eyes, and respiratory system. Is this what you want in your low-calorie diet dessert?

GUILTY OF: Hiding the truth! Because of the labeling loophole, you may not even know that you are ingesting this stuff unless you are reading the ingredients carefully. Neotame is also sold under the name Sweetos as a feed additive for cattle to fatten them up. Sweetos can cover up the smell of the rancid foods often fed to factory-farmed cattle. This is just another great reason to choose grass-fed beef.

Saccharrin

KNOWN ALIASES: Sweet'N Low, Sugar Twin, and E954 (European Union)

RECENT SIGHTINGS: Not used as often as it previously was but still found in many products, including fountain drinks. You can also find it in many over-the-counter medicines, such as Orajel, Scope mouthwash, Mylanta, and Maalox.

SUSPECTED OF: This granddaddy of all the sugar substitutes has a spotted past. Due to allegations that it caused cancer, it was previously removed from products. But now, twenty years later, thanks to relaxed vigilance by both government and consumers (original studies were done on animals, not humans), saccharrin is free to haunt your grocery store aisles once again. The safety of saccharin is still very much in doubt, so steer clear of this potential carcinogenic criminal.

GUILTY OF: Studies by the National Institutes of Health show that rats fed saccharin weighed 20 percent more than rats fed sugar after only five weeks. The sugar substitute did not cause body temperatures to rise, signifying that the body was expending little to no energy (burning calories) to process the foods containing saccharin. Don't let this sugar substitute sabotage your diet plan.

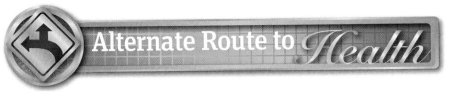

If sugar is an EMD, and Splenda and Sweet'N Low are suspect, what do we suggest? Skip ahead to Aisle 7: Baking to find out.

• • • • • • • • • • • • • • • • • •

Counterfeit Colors

WE EAT WITH OUR EYES as much as with our mouths . . . maybe more. Recent studies have shown that when food manufacturers left foods in their natural (often beige-like) colors instead of coloring them, individuals thought they tasted bland and ate less, even when the recipes had not been altered. How cheesy are beige Cheetos? Is it okay for a strawberry Popsicle to be white? Color often overrides the other parts of the eaters' experience, increasing their appetites when foods appear more vibrant. This explains the food industry's desire to intensify the colors of our foods. The more visually appealing they are, the

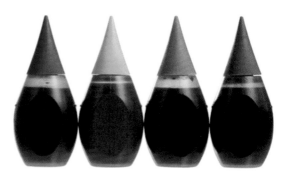

more we will crave them. However, this need to mess with Mother Nature carries with it some very unappetizing side effects.

Until the twentieth century, food coloring was obtained from natural sources. People gathered spices, like saffron and turmeric, to add rich hues to their otherwise bland-colored foods. While this method may have been somewhat limiting in shades, at least it was safe. Today, most artificial colors are made from coal tar. Not familiar with this fine product? Coal tar is also used in sealcoating products to preserve and protect the shine of industrial floors. It also appears in head lice shampoos to kill off the small bugs. From your morning yogurt to your child's cupcake sprinkles, most every food manufactured contains coal tar in the form of artificial colors.

According to the FDA, the increase in processed foods has caused a five-fold increase in consumption of artificial dyes since 1955. Three dyes—red #40, yellow #5, and yellow #6—account for 90 percent of all dyes used. While still approved for use in the United States, many other countries have banned these chemical coloring agents. Here are a couple of the worst offenders to watch out for:

Citrus Red 2

This product caused bladder tumors in animal studies and is banned for human consumption, except to color the skin of oranges. While it may appear to pose little threat, adding fresh orange zest to a recipe may mix in more than you bargained for.

Blue #1 (E133) and Blue #2 (E132)

Banned in Norway, Finland, and France, studies have shown them to cause brain cancer and inhibit nerve-cell development. FOUND IN: *Candy, cereal, soft drinks, sports drinks, and pet food.*

Red #3 (E127) and Red #40 (E129)

While red #3 was banned in 1990 for topical use, it can still be sold on the market in our foods and beverages. That should make us all red in the face. Red #40 may contain the carcinogenic contaminant p-Cresidine and is thought to cause tumors of the immune system. In the UK, it is not recommended for children, and it is currently banned in many European nations. **FOUND IN:** *Fruit cocktail, maraschino cherries, grenadine, cherry pie mix, ice cream, candy, bakery products, and more.*

Yellow #5 (aka Tartazine, E102)

Banned in Norway and Austria, it contains the cancer-causing compounds benzidine and 4-aminobiphenyl. Six of the eleven studies on yellow #5 showed that it caused genotoxicity, a deterioration of the cell's genetic material with potential to mutate healthy DNA. **FOUND IN:** *Gelatin dessert, candy, pet food, and baked goods.*

Yellow #6 (E110)

Banned in Norway and Finland. Due to the same cancer-causing compounds as yellow #5, it causes tumors in the kidneys and adrenal glands of laboratory animals. **FOUND IN:** *American cheese, macaroni and cheese, candy, and carbonated beverages.*

. . . .

Rainbow-Colored Risks

ARE YOUR KIDS CRAZY for colorful foods? Research has associated food dyes with problems in children, including allergies, hyperactivity, learning impairment, irritability, and aggressiveness. A US study published in *Science* found that when children with high scores on a scale measuring hyperactivity consumed a food-dye blend, they performed more poorly on tests that measured their ability to recall images than when given a placebo. A 2007 British study found that within an hour of consuming a mixture of common synthetic dyes, children displayed hyperactive behavior. (These children had not been diagnosed with ADD or ADHD.) The results, published in *The Lancet,* prompted Britain's Food Standards Agency to encourage manufacturers to find alternatives to food dyes. In July 2010, the European Parliament's mandate that foods and beverages containing food dyes must be labeled went into effect for the entire European Union.

Due to the European Union's strong stance against food dyes, many manufacturers have removed them from their products. Nestle, Kraft, Mars, Kellogg's, and even McDonalds all sell their products free of these counterfeit colorings in the EU, proving that there is no need to add these potential poisons into the processed, packaged foods. Until US consumers demand that food manufacturers use natural food dyes, read labels carefully and avoid all products with artificial colors in the ingredient list. We applaud both Trader Joe's and Whole Foods for not allowing any synthetic sinners onto their store shelves.

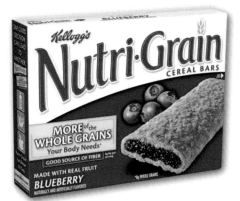 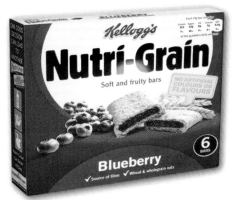

US ingredients: Red #40, Blue #1.   UK ingredients: Beetroot red, Annatto, Paprika extract.

An example of just how easy it is for Kellogg's to replace the synthetic dyes used in the United States with natural colors for their UK products.

• • • • • • • • • • • • • • •

Criminal Chameleons

THESE NEXT TWO INGREDIENTS are tricky. While you may never see their names on the ingredient list, they are often lurking inside.

MSG

While you may know to avoid mono sodium glutamate (MSG) in your Chinese food takeout, you may not be aware that this same flavor enhancer is found in *almost all* processed and packaged foods. This first criminal chameleon's most common side effects are changes in blood pressure, joint pain, diarrhea, blurred vision, irregular heartbeat, depression, an inability to talk, anxiety or panic attacks, migraines, and seizures. However, it is classified as an excitotoxin because the G in MSG (which stands for glutamate or glutamic acid) can cross the blood-brain barrier, overexciting the nerves and causing them to malfunction. Drinking alcohol in conjunction with consuming MSG further compromises the blood-brain barrier and makes it much easier for free glutamate to cause its negative effects. As far back as the 1950s, we already knew that a single dose of MSG could destroy the neurons in the inner layer of a rat's retinas and severely damage the hypothalamus of the brain. **Here is the kicker: studies show that humans are up to six times more sensitive to the effects of MSG than rats!**

Even if you are going to overlook the possible brain damage and the host of other nasty side effects listed above, you still have another reason to avoid MSG. MSG can actually cause you to pack on the pounds. First, it stimulates tastes buds, making bland or even spoiled foods more appetizing. Scientists in Spain found that mice injected with MSG increased their food intake by more than 40 percent. MSG also works to induce obesity because it seems to make us leptin resistant. Recall that leptin is the hormone that makes us feel satiated. Why would you ever put down the chips if your brain never gets the message to stop eating them?

The final way MSG works to supersize us is one that may help to explain the rise in the diabetes epidemic. This ingredient causes the pancreas to secrete insulin, which drops your blood sugar and makes you hungrier faster. When the body over releases insulin, it can lead to insulin resistance, which is the start of type 2 diabetes, heart disease, and many other health problems. MSG-induced obesity is an accepted concept in scientific circles, so much so that when studies require obese animals, the first thing they are fed to fatten them up is MSG.

Processed food manufacturers just love it when you can't stop with a single serving. This is why MSG is so prevalent in Poor Foods throughout your grocery store. According to Vanderbilt University, when food ingredients are listed as "hydrolyzed," "protein fortified," "ultra pasteurized," "fermented," or "enzyme modified," they are often synonymous with MSG, as free glutamic acid is created during processing.

This criminal can be quite a chameleon. We will alert you when mono sodium glutamate may be masquerading under the following aliases: glutamic acid, glutamate, autolyzed yeast, autolyzed yeast protein, yeast extract, textured protein, monopotassium glutamate, calcium glutamate, monoammonium glutamate, magnesium glutamate, sodium caseinate, hydrolyzed corn, yeast food, carrageenan, pectin, soy sauce, and natural flavors.

According to Dr. Cate Shanahan, author of *Deep Nutrition,* 95 percent of all products that boast "natural flavors" contain MSG.

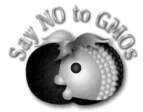

Genetically Modified Organisms (GMOs)

This second chameleon is no less tricky. In fact, unlike MSG, which will occasionally appear on the ingredient list, GMOs are not listed there. Scientists genetically modify crops in order to improve a plant's resistance to pests, make them heartier to survive changes in weather, increase yield, and reduce maturation time. Genetically modifying food takes place in a laboratory when genes from bacteria, viruses, insects, animals, or even humans are artificially inserted into the DNA of food crops or animals. But the health consequences of mating a tomato with a fish, or any other combination that nature has (in its infinite wisdom) forbidden are largely unknown. In fact, not a single human clinical trial on the effects of GMO crops has ever been published. "The experiments simply haven't been done, and we now have become the guinea pigs," said Canadian geneticist David Suzuki. "Anyone that says, 'Oh, we know that this is perfectly safe,' I say is either unbelievably stupid or deliberately lying."

The few animal studies done using GMOs don't look too promising, and scientists worry as to how our bodies will be affected by these unknown mutant genes. Female rats fed GMO soybeans gave birth to stunted and sterile pups. Monarch butterflies, an endangered species, died by the thousands when their favorite food, milkweed, was dusted with GMO corn pollen. Rats fed GMO potatoes developed liver atrophy, damaged hearts, and compromised white blood cell function after only ten days. In Japan, protein shakes made from genetically modified amino acids could not be recalled fast enough, as these never before tested beverages caused metabolic and mental damage to hundreds of men and women—as well as several deaths. Evidence also suggests that the genetic abnormalities of GMO foods may alter the bacteria in the human gut, thereby exposing people to detrimental effects long after a food has been consumed.

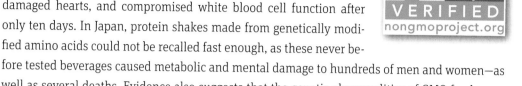

Even with all of these possible negative implications, it may surprise you to see just how prevalent GMOs are in our food supply today. In fact, 80 percent of all packaged processed foods in the grocery store today contain genetically modified ingredients. What's more, the Environmental Working Group reports that while the average American only weighs 179 pounds, he eats a whopping 193 pounds of genetically engineered food a year! This is more than his weight in potentially harmful GMO ingredients annually. Not sure how this affects you? Take a moment to look at the following list of the most common genetically modified foods, and consider how much you are putting yourself at risk.

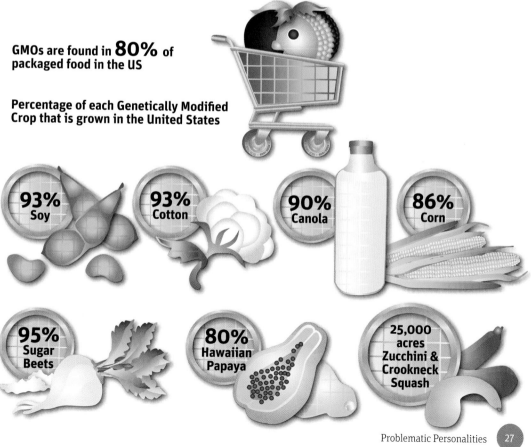

GMOs are found in **80%** of packaged food in the US

Percentage of each Genetically Modified Crop that is grown in the United States

93% Soy

93% Cotton

90% Canola

86% Corn

95% Sugar Beets

80% Hawaiian Papaya

25,000 acres Zucchini & Crookneck Squash

If ubiquitous GMOs aren't bad enough, more than thirty other crops are currently being tested in field trials, including apples, barley, bell peppers, cabbage, carrots, cauliflower, cherries, chili peppers, coffee, cranberries, cucumber, flax, grapefruit, kiwi, lentils, lettuce, melons, mustard, oats, olives, onions, peanuts, pears, peas, persimmons, pineapple, popcorn, radishes, strawberries, sugar cane, sunflower, sweet potatoes, tomatoes, walnuts, and watercress. An excess of forty countries, including China and Japan, require the labeling of genetically modified foods, yet the United States does not. Here are some tips to help you minimize your exposure to GMOs:

1	**Buy USDA-certified organic whenever possible.**
2	**If a product is not organic, look for packages labeled "Non GMO."**
3	**Choose organic or local, pasture-raised dairy and meat to avoid GMO-filled animal feed.**
4	**Avoid at-risk ingredients and their derivatives: soy (soybean oil, soy protein, soy lecithin, vegetable oil), corn (corn oil, HFCS, maltodextrin, cornstarch), canola or rapeseed (canola oil), sugar from sugar beets, cotton (cottonseed oil), zucchini, crooked neck squash, Hawaiian papayas, conventional dairy, meat, and farm-raised fish (most conventional factory-farmed animals eat GMO feed).**
5	**Buy products that are saying no to GMOs. See the appendix Say No to GMOs for a list of companies that keep genetically modified organisms out of their ingredients.**

Note: In our attempt to alert you of possible GMO-sourced ingredients, we have included the letters GMO next to ingredients in our STEER CLEAR selections that we feel have a high likelihood of exposing you to GMOs. We have not, however (as there is no way to know for sure until labeling is required), verified each product individually to be free of GMOs.

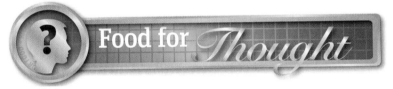

Recently (2012), Californians went to the polls to vote on Proposition 37, which would have required manufacturers to label food products that contained GMOs. Unfortunately, perhaps due to illegal advertising on the part of the pro-GMO lobbyists, it failed, leaving hundreds of millions of unaware Americans vulnerable to the negative health effects of GMOs every time they go grocery shopping. This means that, for now, it is up to each and every one of us to be vigilant and read labels carefully to avoid these Poor Food perpetrators. You can fight back by using your purchasing power to send a clear message to the stores and manufacturers that you will not buy products that contain GMOs. Join the Rich Food Revolution and say no to GMOs!

This GPS is programmed to help you avoid EMDs, sidestep the SSS, and circumvent both the counterfeit colors and criminal chameleons. But we're not out of the woods yet. Keep your eyes peeled for a few more unsavory characters just around the bend.

Chapter 3

Villainous Variables

Jumping right in, we meet three additional groups of Poor Food perpetrators we call the Banned Bad Boys, Label Losers, and Misleading Misfits. Here again, we've already programmed your GPS to avoid them, so there is no need to memorize the numerous ingredients that you are about to uncover. By chapter's end, you will have discovered more than you ever thought possible about your food and will be ready to put that knowledge into practice.

The Banned Bad Boys

WHILE OTHER GOVERNMENTS have read the research and returned guilty verdicts, the United States still allows for the use of the following problematic products. Beware of these bad boys that others have banned!

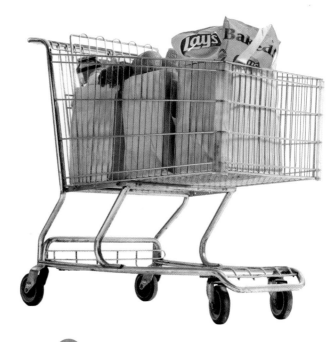

Olestra (aka Olean)

It took the Procter & Gamble Company a quarter century and half a billion dollars to develop its Olestra fat substitute, but it didn't take long for many countries, including the UK and Canada, to ban it. This fat substitute causes a dramatic depletion of fat-soluble vitamins and carotenoids. This makes Olestra an actual EMD, robbing us of the vital micronutrients that our foods should be delivering. However, this bad boy takes it to the next level by actually causing severe gastrointestinal disturbances. While adding Olestra to the ingredients may make your chips "light," it may also cause embarrassing bathroom fright. FOUND IN: *Ruffles Light, Lay's WOW, and Pringles fat-ree potato chips.*

Brominated Vegetable Oil (aka BVO)

Did you have a tough workout? Did your son exhaust himself scoring those goals at his soccer game? It may be time to replenish depleted electrolytes with a thirst-quenching Gatorade. Our guess is that you probably won't be doing much of that after we tell you about one of Gatorade's dirty little ingredients—brominated vegetable oil. BVO acts as an emulsifier in soda and sports beverages, preventing the flavoring from separating and floating to the surface.

BVO is an EMD due to its competition with iodine for receptor sites in the body, causing what is called a brominated thyroid. Elevated bromide levels have been implicated in every thyroid disease, from simple hypothyroidism to autoimmune diseases to thyroid cancer. However, simply stripping your body of an essential micronutrient that so many people are already deficient in isn't BVO's only sin.

This bad boy is composed mainly of bromine, a poisonous chemical whose vapors are considered both corrosive and toxic. BVO is banned in more than one hundred countries. In the United States, its use is regulated by the FDA to the extent that it is "PERMITTED IN FOOD OR IN CONTACT WITH FOOD ON AN INTERIM BASIS PENDING ADDITIONAL STUDY." It doesn't sound like our government is too sure of its safety, either. This may be because BVO has been linked to major organ system damage, birth defects, growth problems, schizophrenia, and hearing loss. FOUND IN: *Mountain Dew, Gatorade, Crush, Sun Drop, Squirt, and Fresca.*

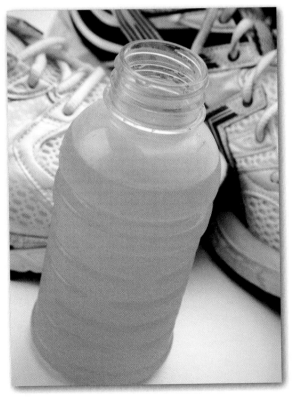

Potassium Bromate (aka Bromated Flour)

Do you notice anything familiar about the name *potassium bromate?* That's right—it is made of the same toxic chemical, bromine, as brominated vegetable oil. This hazardous flour-bulking EMD strengthens dough, decreasing the time needed for baking and thereby reducing costs. This product is harmful because it may cause kidney or nervous system disorders and gastrointestinal discomfort. Additionally, it may be carcinogenic.

The good news is that American bread manufacturers tell us that it disappears from the product during baking and deem that potassium bromate is safe as there is only *negligible residue.* However, the pastry chefs in Paris disagree. In fact, government regulatory bodies in Europe, Canada, China, and many other regions have banned the use of this additive. In California, if potassium bromate has been added, a product must carry a warning label. While the FDA has not banned the use of bromated flour, they do urge bakers to voluntarily leave it out. FOUND IN: *Baja burrito wraps, Jason bread crumbs, Mastroianni Bros rolls, and New York Brands flatbreads and bagel chips.*

Azodicarbonamide

This chemical, whose name just rolls right off the tongue, is banned in Australia, the UK, and most European countries. In Singapore, you can get up to fifteen years in prison and fined nearly half a million dollars for using it as an ingredient. But here, in the good old US of A, we use this chemical that is primarily used in foamed plastics (think yoga mats and sneaker soles) to bleach flour. In other countries, they have to wait a whole week for flour to naturally whiten. Not here! Instead, we add this asthma-causing allergen to numerous grocery store ingredient lists. Examine the labels closely on breads and baked goods before putting them in your cart. FOUND IN: *Stroehmann's breads, Betty Crocker Suddenly Salads, Country Hearth breads, Hungry Man dinners, and Entenmann's baked goods.*

The Butylated Brothers—Butylated Hydroxyanisole or E320 (BHA) and Butylated Hydroxytoluene or E321 (BHT)

Manufactured from petroleum (yummy!), these waxy solids act as preservatives to prevent food from becoming rancid and developing objectionable odors. The National Institutes of Health reports that BHA is reasonably anticipated to be a human carcinogen based on evidence of carcinogenicity in rats. The state of California lists this ingredient as a carcinogen. Banned in England, many other European countries, and Japan, BHA and BHT can be found in butter, meats, breakfast cereals, chewing gum, dehydrated potatoes, and beer sold in the United States. FOUND IN: *Post, Kellogg's, and Quaker cereals; Chex Mix; Diamond nuts; and Wrigley's, Trident, Bazooka, and Bubble Yum chewing gums.*

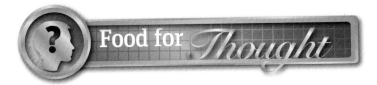

In a 2006 study, the essential oils from natural rosemary and sage performed better at preventing oxidative decay and loss in meat than a combination of BHA and BHT. Perhaps manufacturers should be adding in organic herbs and spices instead of carcinogens to improve the shelf life of their products.

Banned for the Bovines

Recombinant bovine growth hormone (rBGH) and recombinant bovine somatotropin (rBST) are time-saving, production-boosting miracles to steer clear of. Dairy farmers in the United States commonly inject cows with genetically engineered bovine (cow) growth hormones, sold under the trade name Posilac, in order to boost milk production by about 10 percent. However, several regions, including Australia, New Zealand, Canada, Japan, and the European Union, have banned rbGH and rBST because of their dangerous impacts on both human and bovine health.

Cows treated with these synthetic hormones often become lame, infertile, and suffer from inflamed and infected breasts (udders). Humans fare no better. The unnatural milk is supercharged with IGF-1 (insulin growth factor -1). This nearly 70 percent increase in IGF-1 is readily absorbed through the gut and has been linked to breast, colon, and prostate cancers. Buying organic milk, and milk labeled rBGH/rBST-free, is your best bet for avoiding cows treated with these controversial chemicals.

The following national brands are produced without rBGH:

- Alta Dena
- Belgioioso Cheese Inc.
- Ben & Jerry's Ice Cream
- Brown Cow Farm
- Crowley Cheese of Vermont
- Franklin County Cheese
- Grafton Village Cheese
- Great Hill Dairy
- Lifetime Dairy
- Nancy's Natural Dairy
- Roth Kase USA
- Walmart store brand
- Yoplait

Label Losers

WHILE THESE INGREDIENTS have not been banned, your GPS has been programmed to avoid these violators as well. Some act as EMDs and others bring with them some unwanted health risks. Minimizing their presence in your cart will maximize the quality of your food.

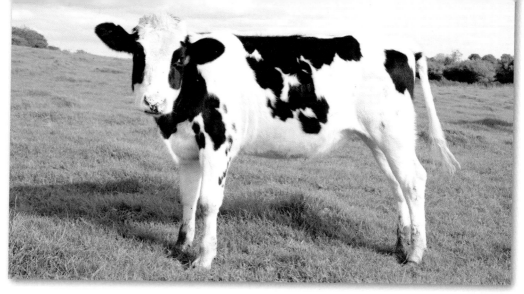

Ammonium Sulfate

Most commonly used as a fertilizer to nourish the garden, it is also used to nourish yeast to turn bread a "healthy" brown color. This dough conditioner may cause mouth ulcers, nausea, and kidney and liver problems.

Benzoates: Sodium Benzoate/Potassium Benzoate

These preservatives extend shelf life by preventing the growth of microorganisms in acidic foods like fruit juices and soda. While they seem to be safe for some, they cause allergic reactions, hives, and asthma in others. The real problem is that when benzoates come in contact with vitamin C (ascorbic acid), they form a known carcinogen called benzene. While the risk may be small, why take it at all?

BPA, Bisphenol-A

While you will never find BPA as a listed food ingredient, this toxic troublemaker must be avoided. BPA is a synthetic estrogen that has been used to package consumer goods since the 1950s. It can be found in reusable drink containers, DVDs, cell phones, eyeglass lenses, and automobile parts. In the grocery store, you are most likely to come in contact with it in polycarbonate plastics used for water bottles and in the lining of food cans. It is even in the thermal paper used for cash register receipts. The BPA used in containers can seep into your food and beverages. BPA is especially good at leaching into canned foods that are acidic, salty, or fatty, such as coconut milk, tomatoes, canned fish, soup, and vegetables. A Center for Disease Control report found BPA in the urine of 93 percent of adults.

According to the Environmental Working Group, "Trace BPA exposure has been shown to disrupt the endocrine system and trigger a wide variety of disorders, including chromosomal and reproductive system abnormalities, impaired brain and neurological functions, cancer, cardiovascular system damage, adult-onset diabetes, early puberty, obesity, and resistance to chemotherapy."

The Food and Drug Administration is concerned and is taking steps to reduce human exposure to BPA in the food supply, so much so that it has banned BPA use in infant bottles. However, until it is removed from all plastics, here are some tips to help you minimize your exposure:

1 Look for products labeled BPA-free*.

2 Choose glass, porcelain, or stainless steel containers over aluminum or plastic bottles, cans, and containers.

3 Don't choose plastic bottles that have the numbers 3 or 7 recycling symbols on the bottom. Number 6 is dangerous as well, but for different reasons.

4 Never microwave in plastic containers.

5 Never wash or reuse plastic containers not labeled as BPA free (e.g., ribbed bottles or water containers).

6 Reduce your use of canned goods unless they are labeled BPA free.*

*Many companies are slowly removing the BPA lining from their cans. Some companies don't use BPA lining but do not label their cans to identify which cans are safe. Therefore, identifying BPA-free canned and bottled products is difficult. Your best bet, and the only true way to be sure, is to call the manufacturer and ask. Here in *Rich Food, Poor Food,* we have made it easy and asked them for you. You can be assured that every canned item in this book has been identified by its manufacturer as BPA free.

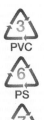

A possible carcinogen. Found in bottles and clear food packaging, number 3 plastics may release toxins into your food and drinks. The risk is heightened when these containers are put through the dishwasher, heated up, or frozen. Flexible plastics may contain BPA as well.

Number 6 plastics are what we call Styrofoam and release toxins into our food when heated up.

Found in baby bottles, water bottles, and food containers, number 7 containers can leach bisphenol A—a hormone disrupter that can lead to neural and behavioral problems in children. BPA is a synthetic hormone that can stimulate premature puberty and even lead to breast development in males. BPA has also been linked to prostate cancer.

Caramel Coloring

This brown coloring agent contains the contaminants 2-methylimidazole and 4-methylimidazole. It can be found in baked goods, pre-cooked meats, soy and Worcestershire sauces, chocolate-flavored products, and beer, but the worst offender of all is cola. This criminal coloring agent is linked to lung, liver, and thyroid cancer.

Carrageenan

This thickening, emulsifying, and stabilizing ingredient started out as red seaweed and can be found in numerous milk beverages, deli meats, and pizza crusts. This gooey additive (often used to de-ice airplanes) has been shown to cause ulcerations and malignancies in the gastrointestinal tract. If that doesn't make you uneasy, then perhaps knowing that it may also contain MSG (see mono sodium glutamate in Chapter 2) may be enough to keep this creep out of the cart.

Ethylenediaminetetraacetic Acid (aka Disodium EDTA)

This synthetic chemical most commonly used for medicinal purposes chelates (binds) to metals in the body to draw them out. While this may be a great medical treatment for heavy metal poisoning, imagine how disturbing it can be to the essential minerals your body needs to function properly. Commonly added to preserve color and flavor in processed foods, this ingredient works as an EMD, depleting your body of vitamin C, magnesium, iron, calcium, zinc, and potassium.

Guar Gum

Similar in function to carrageenan, this emulsifier/thickener made from ground guar beans is used in various products, such as beverages, soups, cottage cheese, and some frozen desserts. Due to guar gum's high levels of soluble fiber, it actually acts as an EMD, significantly reducing the absorption of the carotenoids beta-carotene, lycopene, and lutein.

Pectin

This gelling agent is extracted from citrus fruits and used to thicken jams, jellies, fruit juices, milk drinks, canned frosting, and yogurt. Unlike some of the others on this list, pectin is not toxic or carcinogenic. However, much like guar gum, this gooey fiber acts as an EMD, pulling out important micronutrients (beta-carotene, lycopene, and lutein.) Bottom line: you get much less nutrition than you bargained for.

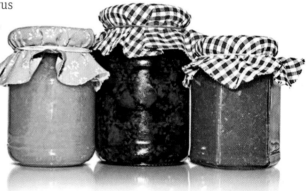

Sodium Nitrite

While this synthetic ingredient does brighten your bacon and preserve your pastrami, when you see sodium nitrite on an ingredient list, it should raise a caution flag in your mind. However, it may not for the reason you once believed. There has long been debate about the safety of sodium nitrite. You probably have been told that eating foods that contain nitrites will cause cancer. However, did you know that your body converts the naturally occurring *nitrates* found in fruits, vegetables, and grains into *nitrites*? In fact, nearly 93 percent of all the nitrates consumed come from non-meat sources! Even celery juice or powder, which often replace the synthetic nitrites in packaged cured meats, has nitrates.

Regardless of the source, when sodium nitrate is consumed, it is converted to sodium nitrite. When these nitrites combine with amines, which are naturally present in meat, N-nitroso compounds, or nitrosamines, are formed. These compounds were once considered carcinogenic because several decades ago, researchers saw a link to cancer in lab rats. That started a media frenzy, which somehow became an urban myth or pseudo-science. It turns out there is no real proof of this connection . . . they were wrong. Indeed, the National Academy of Sciences, the National Research Council, and even the American Cancer Society all agree that there's no cancer risk from consuming sodium nitrite.

Then why did we say that you should be cautious when you see synthetic sodium nitrite? Well, as it turns out, the synthetic sodium nitrite, used to cure meats, may not be that healthy for us for a different reason. According to the Food Chemical Codex (3rd edition, National Academy of Sciences), industrial sodium nitrite (synthetic) is allowed to contain residual heavy metals—arsenic and lead. Thus, our choice to dodge nitrites, in favor of their celery and sea salt natural alternatives, is due not to the media-driven myth of cancer-causing nitrosamines but due to the scientifically documented heavy metal mix-ins.

Partially Hydrogenated Vegetable Oil and Partially Hydrogenated Soybean Oil

When vegetable oil and hydrogen are combined through a process called hydrogenation, it creates a product with greater stability that is less likely to spoil. The product is trans fat, something that, according to Harvard School of Public Health, causes about fifty thousand premature heart attack deaths annually. Beware of this hydrogen bomb ingredient in commercial crackers, cookies, cakes, doughnuts, frozen dinners, and french fries. Shortenings and margarines can also be high in trans fat. This dangerous ingredient has been shown to raise LDL cholesterol and lower HDL cholesterol, increasing the risk of cardiovascular disease and heart attack by 50 percent! Trans fats also increase the risk for obesity, birth defects, insulin resistance, diabetes, depression, asthma, cell damage, osteoporosis, and cancer, especially breast cancer. Even though the National Academy of Science's Institute of Medicine made its recommendation to the FDA way back in 2002 stating that no amount of trans fat in the diet is safe, this Poor Food ingredient is still allowed in our food as long as manufacturers list the amount of trans fats on the Nutrition Facts label.

But don't be fooled. Many processed foods that claim zero grams of this deadly ingredient on the Nutrition Facts still contain trans fats. How? Because the FDA allows food manufacturers to take advantage of a labeling loophole and list zero trans fat on the Nutrition Facts if their food has less than half a gram of trans fat per serving. However, if you see Poor Food ingredients like partially hydrogenated oil, hydrogenated oil, or shortening on the ingredient list, you can be sure that trans fats are still lurking in your food. Even seemingly innocent products like Girl Scout cookies, sold to millions by well-intentioned children, may contain this Franken-fat.

Monoglyceride and Diglyceride

These food additives are labeled as emulsifiers because they allow fats and waters to mix smoothly, which extends the shelf life of processed foods. They are created when hydrogen gas passes through heated hardened palm oil. Sound familiar? They are created much in the same way as our trans fats are created by partially hydrogenating vegetable oil. However, the difference is that partially hydrogenated oil is classified as a lipid (fat), which means that the trans fat must be labeled on a product's package. Even though mono and diglycerides may contain trans-fatty acids, they do not fall under these FDA labeling requirements because they are labeled as emulsifiers, not lipids. This semantics loophole allows food that contains those same trans-fatty acids that have been associated with heart disease, stroke, obesity, and diabetes to be marketed as possessing "0 percent trans fat."

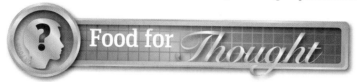

All trans fats are bad, right? Wrong! Did you know that CLA (conjugated linoleic acid)— a natural fat found in grass-fed meat and dairy, pastured eggs, and kangaroo meat—is also a trans fat? CLA has been shown to have numerous health benefits, including fat-burning and anti-cancer properties. It is the synthetically produced trans-fatty acids in partially hydrogenated vegetable oils and mono and diglycerides that are bad. This is just another dangerous example of misinformation that can occur when we try to put the science of nutrition into a neat little box.

Sulfites (Sodium Sulfite, Sulfur Dioxide, Sodium Bisulfite, Calcium Sulphite)

Individuals who suffer from asthma and allergies are warned to steer clear of sulfites, as they can cause anaphylactic shock and have even caused death. However, that's not the only trick up sulfite's sleeve. It also acts as an EMD—destroying thiamin (vitamin B1), a micronutrient needed for mental clarity and heart health. While sulfites are banned in fruits and vegetables, they can still be found in potatoes, shrimp, wine, and beer.

Now, let's redirect our focus from the product's ingredient list to the front of the package or billboard. Here we will find all sorts of claims that act as misleading misfits.

• • • • • • • • • • • • • •

Misleading Misfits

THESE MISLEADING MISFITS may just take you on a trip to the land of broken promises, but it isn't necessarily their fault. The following words and phrases are sanctioned by the FDA and have very specific definitions. The problem comes when we think they mean something other than what they really mean. Less-than-honest food manufacturers often use these enticing words and phrases as billboard bullies—conning you into buying something you really don't want. It's time to unmask these misfits to learn their true identities.

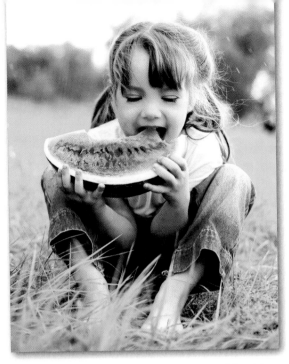

"Natural" and "Fresh"

In the supermarket arena, the word *natural* is the darling of the day. It turns out the word really hits the sweet spot with consumers, even outselling labeled "certified organic" products by more than 2 to 1. Because of this, food companies are rebranding everything to be "natural." So what does *natural* mean? According to the FDA and USDA's Food Safety and Inspection Service (FSIS), products advertised as "natural" should not contain any synthetic or artificial ingredients, and in the case of meat products must be minimally processed. However, they can still contain decidedly unnatural and health-compromising ingredients, such as high fructose corn syrup (HFCS), partially hydrogenated vegetable oil, and modified food starch. Products labeled as "natural" can be produced using hormones, pesticides, antibiotics, chemical fertilizers, genetic engineering, and, yes, sewage sludge! More than fifty million tons of treated sewage sludge removed from drains of homes, business, and industry are spread on farmlands in North Carolina alone every year. More than sixty thousand toxic substances and chemical compounds can be found in the sewage sludge that is being used to fertilize our foods!

Fresh is another word that may not mean what you think. While the FDA demands that "fresh" food is in a raw state and has not been frozen or subjected to any form of thermal processing or preservation, it does allow for the following unappealing processes: waxing or coating, post-harvest pesticides, and a mild chlorine, acid wash, or ionizing radiation (that's irradiation, not to exceed the maximum dose of 1 kiloGray, the equivalent of thirty-three million chest X-rays.) Do you see how a diet of natural, fresh foods may still be damaging to your health?

"Made With" or "Contains"

When you see claims that begin with *made with* or *contains,* it is a good indicator that the manufacturer is trying to bait you into thinking a product is healthier than it is. It is likely that you are buying a product that *contains* or is *made with* more Poor Food ingredients than you bargained for. For example, a Rich Food indicator would be terminology like *100 percent real fruit juice* or *made from only 100 percent real fruit juice.* Can you see the difference? Saying *made with* or *contains* real fruit juice is like claiming *low mileage* on a 1969 Chevy. Low compared with what? Other 1969 Chevys? Saying that the car has 40,000 miles, however, is specific and tells the buyer exactly what he is getting.

Everyone knows that adding real fruit to your diet is a great way to increase health through micronutrient sufficiency. Misleading manufacturers use the phrase *made with real fruit* to increase the chances that consumers looking for healthy products will mistakenly purchase their Poor Food knockoffs. While the billboards claim *real fruit inside,* too often this fruit comes in the form of natural colorings, like beet juice or fruit concentrates, which are really just the pure sugars that supply no health benefits at all. Beware of these claims, and buy whole fruits instead!

"Healthy"

So, what does the FDA think is healthy? You may be surprised to discover that it may not fit into your dietary profile at all. This is because the term *healthy* only relates to the Nutrition Facts on the packaging—that same part of the package that almost tricked us into buying the Baked! Lays. The FDA deems foods that have limited fat, cholesterol, and sodium as healthy, and much like the other swap books, those in packaging power do not consider overall carbohydrate count in this equation. There are many different dietary philosophies that would be left out in the cold using this restrictive definition.

Additionally, these healthy foods can stir anything they want into the list of ingredients and still maintain their "healthy" status. So, a healthy, low-fat, low-sodium fruit cup will meet the requirements, even if MSG has been added to the GMO fruit in a BPA can. Not sure about you, but the word *healthy* seems to be losing the appeal it once had. Make sure to read the ingredient list and use your GPS to find truly healthy Rich Foods.

• • • • • • • • • • • • • • •

Organic

ORGANIC IS ANOTHER WORD you find on many labels that does have a very specific meaning. Here again, though, manufacturers have ways of manipulating the meaning. According to the *USDA Organic Production and Handling Standards,* the term *organic* requires that a food be free of potentially harmful or toxic pesticides, herbicides, chemical fertilizers, sewage sludge, artificial hormones (including recombinant bovine growth hormone—rBGH and rBST), antibiotics, and genetically modified organisms (GMOs). They also demand that food has not been processed using irradiation, chemical food additives, or industrial solvents. Products made with 95 to 100 percent certified organic foods can proudly display the USDA organic seal on their packages.

Then you have the conniving callout that claims it is *made with* organic products. What does this mean? Remember, *made with* also means that some of it is *made without.* When you see *made with* on a label referring to organics, the USDA regulates this to mean that 70 percent of a product is certified organic. This leaves you 30 percent exposed. Still not *so* awful. But then there are the misleading manufacturers that use one or two organic ingredients so the word *organic* pops out when you read the list of ingredients. Just because one or two ingredients are organic does not mean that the rest of the ingredients are. You may drop it into your cart if you aren't paying close attention.

On the whole, any step toward organic is good, but you don't want to pay top dollar for a product that just contains a small amount of organic ingredients when, for the same price, you could have purchased a USDA certified organic product that carries the seal.

Whew! Now that you have learned the lay of the label as well as the numerous EMDs, mischievous mix-ins, villainous variables, and label losers to avoid, you are ready to grab yourself a cart and begin your grocery shopping.

Let the Adventure Begin!

IT'S TIME TO TURN IN YOUR LEARNER'S PERMIT because you've just earned your Rich Food license to shop. Like any new driver, you are bound to hit a few rough patches. However, you now have all the information you need to successfully navigate your grocery store adventure. We guarantee it will be a shopping trip unlike any before! Aisle after aisle, you won't look at food the same way again. Oh, and even though you have the basics down, we will be there with you in each department—from the dairy section to the beverage aisle—to offer you more information and tips for finding the healthiest, most micronutrient-rich foods possible for you and your family.

Most first-time Rich Food shoppers come back as if they had just gone on an African safari. They enthusiastically talk of how they hunted down the Rich Foods and spotted plenty of Poor Foods along the way. Your shopping safari will take you on a guided tour *around* your supermarket—literally. We begin by navigating you along the perimeter of the store. And for good reason—almost all the *real* foods are located there. The interior aisles are like food deserts when it comes to micronutrient values, so we want you to start each shopping trip by filling up as much of your cart as you can with the real, micronutrient-packed Rich Foods along the perimeter of the market. As you learn to emphasize the perimeter, it will become second nature to avoid the highly processed, boxed, bagged, bottled, and canned foods filling the interior shelves.

Additionally, we should warn you that the likelihood of your *first* Rich Food shopping adventure being a quick one is slim to none. Most first-time Rich Food shoppers spend more time than usual identifying the Rich Food choices available in their grocery store, so schedule time for this adventure. A tight schedule, a hungry belly, or a cart full of restless kids will not make for an enjoyable or productive experience. If you are crunched for time, you may choose to tackle only one or two aisles per visit. Rest assured, once you have located your Rich Foods, the time you usually spend shopping will be cut in half, because your research and due diligence will have paid off. So jump to it. Happy shopping!

PART TWO

Ready, Set . . . Shop!

Aisle ONE

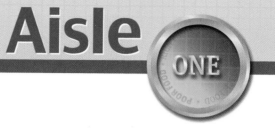

Dairy

When you enter the dairy section of most supermarkets, suddenly the aisles part and the store widens. You find yourself in a brightly lit area, surrounded by softly humming, colossal-size coolers filled with every dairy product imaginable. But which brands should you choose for better health? Do grass-fed cows give more nourishing milk, or are organic milks better? Is there a nutritional difference between block cheese and shredded cheese? With such an array of choices, it can get confusing. No worries—your GPS has been preprogrammed to direct you to our Rich Food choices. So push that cart and begin shopping confidently and healthfully in the dairy section.

The Advantages of Grass-fed and Organic Dairy

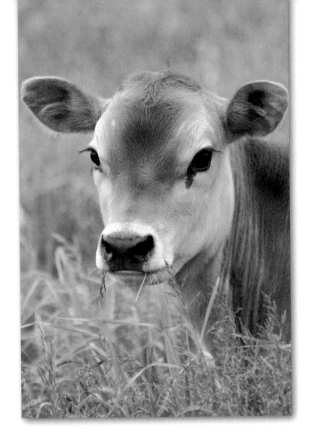

BEFORE WE DELVE INTO DAIRY, it is important to examine two terms used to qualify dairy, from milk to Muenster cheese, yogurt to sour cream. How much do you know about the terms *grass-fed* and *organic*?

Let's first examine the term *grass-fed*. Until about a hundred years ago, cows were given a diet restricted to their native food, grass. However, cost-cutting strategies have created feedlots where the cows are fed grains and stale candy (up to seven pounds a day) to hasten their growth and are no longer allowed to feed naturally on grass.

On your dairy expedition, we advocate consuming often elusive grass-fed products because doing so helps avoid Everyday Micronutrient Depleter #2: Unnatural Feed and Environment *and* because studies show that dairy products from grass-fed cows are better for you. Why? Cows are supposed to eat grass, and when they do, they properly receive all the essential micronutrients and deliver them to you. Grass-fed cows also deliver two fantastic essential fats: conjugated linoleic acid (CLA), which has cancer-fighting and fat-metabolizing potential, and omega-3, which cools inflammation and is thought to reduce the risk of cancer and cardiovascular disease. The bottom line is that healthy grass-fed cows produce healthy micronutrient-rich milk, cheese, yogurt, and butter. However, the term *grass-fed* can't tell us anything more. It begins and ends with what the cattle has been fed. It cannot tell you if the grass the cow is fed is from GMO seeds, if it has been sprayed with pesticides, or if it has been grown using synthetic fertilizer. It also cannot guarantee you that the animal has not been give antibiotics or synthetic hormones. Read grass-fed on the label like this:

GRASS-FED

This animal has been fed only grass, no grains

When you see *organic* on a dairy label, it means something altogether different than *grass-fed*. According to the *USDA Organic Produc-*

tion and Handling Standards, the term *organic* requires that cows be unconfined and allowed to eat grass for the entire grazing season (not less than 120 days) and that at least 30 percent of their feed or dry matter intake must be from grasses. This leaves 70 percent of their food potentially coming from grains. While some studies have shown that organic foods, including dairy products, contain higher levels of micronutrients, the true benefit of organic foods is their ability to protect from potentially harmful toxins. Organic cattle receive no synthetic hormones or antibiotics, and the 70 percent of time they are not eating grasses, organic cattle must be given feed that is free of GMOs, pesticides, and synthetic fertilizers.

So, as we move through the dairy section, look for products that are organic *and* grass-fed, so that you are protected from harmful exposure while enjoying the most nutritional benefits from your dairy products.

GRASS-FED

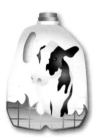

WHAT IT IS:

100 percent grass-fed

WHAT IT IS NOT

Hormone free

Antibiotic free

Free of GMOs in feed

Free of pesticides in feed

Free of feed grown in
synthetic fertilizer

ORGANIC

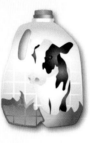

WHAT IT IS:

Hormone free

Antibiotic free

Free of GMOs in feed

Free of pesticides in feed

Free of feed grown in
synthetic fertilizer

WHAT IT IS NOT:

100 percent grass-fed

ORGANIC GRASS-FED

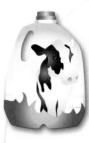

WHAT IT IS:

100 percent grass-fed

Hormone free

Antibiotic free

Free of GMOs in feed

Free of pesticides in feed

Free of feed grown in synthetic fertilizer

WHAT IT IS NOT:

Easy to find—until enough people demand it

DAIRY

Food for *Thought*

Don't be duped by dairy products claiming that cows are pastured. While some farmers may be using the term *pastured* to mean *grass-fed*, the USDA does not regulate this claim. The dairy may not deliver all the nutritional benefits of grass-fed dairy because while the cows might have visited a pasture or two, the majority of their diet could still have consisted of grain.

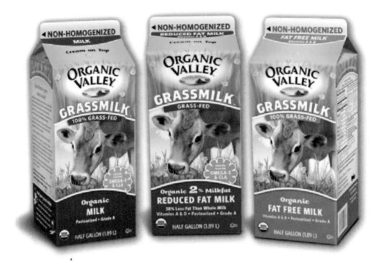

Milk

Milk is packaged based on the percentage of fat it contains, but this is not a factor we consider when choosing our Rich Food milk choices. In fact, the hierarchy of milk products we have outlined in this aisle hold true across the board, from skim milk to heavy cream. While many health-conscious consumers stridently believe that skim milk is better than 2 percent, which is better than whole milk, this assertion is debatable. Low-carb and evolutionary health devotees will recommend whole milk to provide more satiating fats and limit exposure to carbs, which are consumed in excess with the Standard American Diet. Whatever your personal preference of milk, our goal is to direct you to the healthiest option, regardless of its fat and calorie count.

Pasteurization: the Destruction of Raw Milk

THE METHOD OF PREPARING MILK for sale has changed dramatically, much like the changes in the raising and feeding of cattle, which we will discuss in Aisle 2: Meat, but it wasn't so long ago that everyone drank fresh, natural, unpasteurized (raw) milk. However, due to some unsanitary urban farms back in the 1800s, a temporary solution called pasteurization was implemented. It turned out that pasteurization was a lot more cost effective than maintaining clean farms. When large dairy farms saw the potential for mass production and increased profits using the new "cleaning" technique, they never looked back.

Pasteurization, our Everyday Micronutrient Depleter #3, is a heat treatment that kills bacteria. Not only does pasteurization kill the friendly bacteria (yes, there are some bacteria that are good for us, like probiotics), it greatly diminishes milk's natural micronutrient content. Milk, in its unpasteurized, natural state, is full of essential micronutrients, including vitamins A, D, B6, B12, calcium, and CLA.

The process of pasteurization, and especially ultra-pasteurization, denatures—alters the original molecular structure of the proteins in the milk itself. These new flattened molecules can pass easily into the bloodstream, causing an increasingly common health condition called leaky gut syndrome. When these denatured proteins enter the intestinal tract where they do not belong, they are perceived as foreign, and the body mounts an immune response. This can lead to an overstressed immune system, reduced micronutrient absorption, gastrointestinal problems, and chronic fatigue.

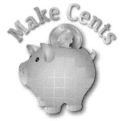

Don't waste your money on ultra-pasteurized organic milk. Ultra-pasteurization heats milk to an even higher temperature, further extending its shelf life and further damaging its protein structure. While this may allow for maximum fridge time, it contains minimal micronutrients. Check labels when purchasing organic milk, and steer clear of this micronutrient depleter.

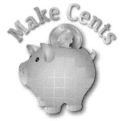DAIRY

Homogenized Milk and Heart Health

IN ADDITION TO BEING PASTEURIZED, the majority of the milk in the supermarket is homogenized. Most people are familiar with this term but unaware of the potential health hazards of this process.

Homogenization is the process of forcing milk under extreme pressure through tiny holes in order to break up the normally large fat particles into smaller ones. This is done so that the cream, which normally rests at the top of the milk container, is denatured to form smaller molecular clusters that stay suspended within the milk itself.

The cream still remains in the milk, but homogenization fundamentally changes the way the body digests and absorbs it. Here's how. The smaller particles make absorption of the fat and proteins across the gut wall much easier and quicker. This in turn can increase the occurrences and severity of allergic reactions in some people.

Mary G. Enig, PhD, of the Weston A Price Foundation explains it this way: "During homogenization, there is a tremendous increase in surface area on the fat globules. The original fat globule membrane is lost, and a new one is formed that incorporates a much greater portion of casein and whey proteins. This may account for the increased allergenicity of modern processed milk."

So, perhaps the slogan, "Milk—it does the body good," might be amended to: "Traditional non-homogenized, unpasteurized raw milk—it does the body good."

D-licious!

VITAMIN D HAS BEEN TOUTED the skinny vitamin because studies have shown that women sufficient in this powerful, fat-soluble vitamin weigh, on average, 16.3 pounds less than those deficient. Pretty amazing, right? Additionally, vitamin D has been shown to aid in the prevention of cancer, heart disease, type 2 diabetes, and depression. The best source of vitamin D is the sun. A typical summer session in a bathing suit can supply an incredible 10,000 IU of this health-promoting micronutrient. However, individuals with darker skin, those working through the midday hours, and the masses living during the winter months on a latitude north of Atlanta (approximately 33 degrees north) may find themselves unable to reap the benefits of sunbathing. These individuals need to take a vitamin D supplement and search out food sources to stay sufficient.

Almost all milk is fortified with vitamin D (approximately 100 IU, or 25 percent of your recommended daily intake) to help the absorption of calcium, which is essential for strong teeth and bones. However, not all forms of vitamin D act the same in your body. Unless you are a vegan or strict vegetarian, we recommend you choose a brand that contains vitamin D3 (animal based) rather than D2 (from plant/yeast) because studies show D3 is the preferred vitamin source for humans and has been found to be more effective at delivering health benefits than D2.

Adding in a Little O?

BY NOW, MOST OF US have heard of omega-3 and its fantastic health benefits, including brain function, heart health, and anti-inflammation. So it's no surprise that many brands are now adding this essential fatty acid into their milk—and their labels. Farm-fresh, unpasteurized, raw milk already has increased levels of omega-3 fatty acids, but if we are buying a factory-farmed, pasteurized carton of milk, it makes sense to choose one that gives you an added omega-3 boost. However, again, unless you are vegan or a strict vegetarian, we recommend that the milk you choose lists actual fish oil rather than DHA from an algae source. This is because fish oil supplies EPA *and* DHA, which are both important to your overall health, while algae-sourced omega-3 supplies only DHA.

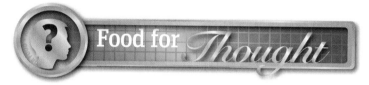

Food for *Thought*

According to research done at Cornell University Department of Food Science, milk packaged in opaque or cardboard cartons contains more micronutrients than milk in clear jugs or bottles. This is because vitamin A is sensitive to light, and when researchers examined the amount of vitamin A loss in whole, 2 percent, and fat-free milk, they found that up to 20 percent of the vitamin A in fat-free milk was lost after just two hours of fluorescent light exposure similar to the lighting in a grocery store. After sixteen hours, the fat-free milk lost nearly 55 percent of its vitamin A content. Whole milk and 2 percent fared much better due to their higher fat content, which protects vitamin A, losing only 10 percent and 25 percent, respectively, after sixteen hours. Vitamin C and vitamin B2 (riboflavin) are also sensitive to light and are greatly reduced in milk exposed to light.

Got Goat?

HAVE MILK ALLERGIES? Maybe goat milk is the answer you have been looking for. According to the *Journal of American Medicine,* it's the most complete food known, containing vitamins, minerals, electrolytes, trace elements, enzymes, protein, and fatty acids that are utilized by the body with ease. In fact, your body can digest goat's milk in just twenty minutes, compared with the two to three hours it takes for your body to digest cow's milk. Goat's milk has higher levels of fat-metabolizing CLA and inflammation-fighting omega-3 than cow's milk and supplies twice as much of the electrolyte potassium. Additionally, according to Texas A&M University, goat's milk has more acid-buffering capacity than nonprescription antacid drugs. Due to goat milk's lower levels of lactose (a form of sugar found in milk), individuals who are lactose intolerant (or who produce an

DAIRY

inadequate amount of lactase, an enzyme required for the digestion of lactose) prefer it. Also, it is extra high in selenium—a micronutrient important for the prevention of cancer and diabetes.

Lactose-Free Milk

WHILE GOAT'S MILK MAY BE a relief for some, many people can't tolerate any kind of milk. This could be due to a milk allergy or serious lactose intolerance. According to the National Institutes of Health (NIH), lactose intolerance is estimated to affect thirty to fifty million Americans. If you are one of them, you may want to consider lactose-free milk. While no milk comes out of a cow or goat lactose free, manufacturers add lactate to the milk to predigest the lactose for you, making milk that is virtually free of lactose. The great news is that it looks and tastes the same as regular milk, but it doesn't cause stomach upset in lactose-intolerant individuals.

If you still get stomach upset or other reactions with lactose-free milk, you may have a milk allergy or may be having a reaction to the denatured proteins present in all pasteurized milk. Pasteurization also destroys the lactase that is naturally found in unpasteurized milk, the enzyme we just learned is necessary for the digestion of the lactose in milk. It may actually be the pasteurization process itself that is causing the intolerance. To find out for sure, you may want to try unpasteurized raw milk. For many people, farm-fresh raw milk solves their milk miseries.

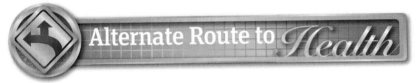

You may not be surprised to learn that our #1 Rich Food choice for milk cannot be purchased in most grocery stores. Yep, you guessed it—it's farm-fresh, grass-fed, unpasteurized, and non-homogenized (raw) milk. We think it is the "cream of the crop" because, as we have just learned, it is far richer in vitamins, minerals, essential fatty acids, and healthy bacteria than its factory-farmed, pasteurized (heated) or ultra-pasteurized (highly heated), and homogenized, denatured, micronutrient-depleted counterparts. We feel it's worth going the extra mile (or twenty) to a local farm to get it. BUYER BEWARE: Unpasteurized milk can cause serious illness if not handled properly. Make sure to inspect the cleanliness of the farm from which you buy it.

As we outlined in *Naked Calories,* there are numerous micronutrient benefits to choosing natural, raw, grass-fed milk for your fridge. Here are just a few:

- Up to 60 percent more thiamine (vitamin B1) and B6 than pasteurized milk
- Up to 100 percent more B12
- Up to 30 percent more folate (vitamin B9)
- Increased amounts of both calcium and phosphorus
- Contains vitamin K2, greater amounts of CLA, and healthy omega-3s

DO PEOPLE IN OTHER COUNTRIES DRINK NATURAL (RAW) MILK?

YOU BET THEY DO! In fact, in France, Slovenia, and Poland, raw milk is sold on the streets out of dispenser machines, similar to our soda and vending machines, called mlekomats (milk–o–mats—get it?!). In Italy, these *moo-chines* are called latterias. Raw, non-pasteurized, non-homogenized milk is the milk of our grandparents, their parents, and *their* parents— all the way back to the beginning of time.

Drinking this milk is common in many regions, including Africa, India, Asia, New Zealand, and the twenty-seven member states of the European Union. The UK even has twenty-four-hour raw milk delivery.

To find a local farmer that sells rich, raw milk and to learn more about individual state laws, go to: CaltonNutrition.com/ Rich-Food.

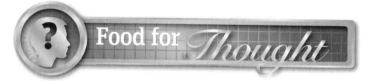

Food for *Thought*

Many cereals today are fortified with numerous vitamins and minerals to help you start your day off right. Have you ever wondered whether your body is really absorbing them? If you pour skim milk or a low-fat milk substitute into your cereal bowl, you may be defeating the purpose. Fat-soluble vitamins like A, D, E, and K are just as essential to your body as the water-soluble vitamins like vitamin C and the many B vitamins. However, for them to be optimally absorbed, your body *needs* fat. So, if you are eating a low-fat or fat-free cereal fortified with these fat-soluble vitamins, using a milk option with a higher fat content may be beneficial to assist the absorption of those vitamins. For Rich Food cereal options, visit Aisle 6: Grains.

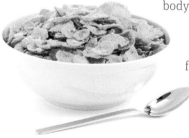

DAIRY

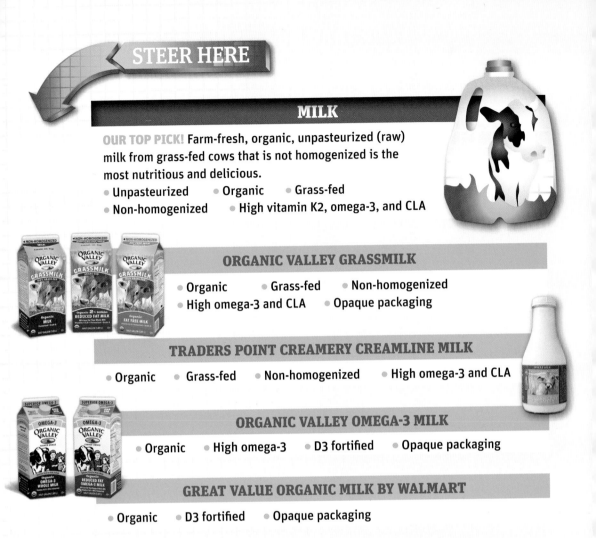

STEER HERE

MILK

OUR TOP PICK! Farm-fresh, organic, unpasteurized (raw) milk from grass-fed cows that is not homogenized is the most nutritious and delicious.
- Unpasteurized
- Organic
- Grass-fed
- Non-homogenized
- High vitamin K2, omega-3, and CLA

ORGANIC VALLEY GRASSMILK
- Organic
- Grass-fed
- Non-homogenized
- High omega-3 and CLA
- Opaque packaging

TRADERS POINT CREAMERY CREAMLINE MILK
- Organic
- Grass-fed
- Non-homogenized
- High omega-3 and CLA

ORGANIC VALLEY OMEGA-3 MILK
- Organic
- High omega-3
- D3 fortified
- Opaque packaging

GREAT VALUE ORGANIC MILK BY WALMART
- Organic
- D3 fortified
- Opaque packaging

CREAM

NATURAL BY NATURE GRASS-FED HEAVY CREAM
- Organic
- Grass-fed
- Non-homogenized
- High omega-3 and CLA
- Opaque packaging

GOAT MILK

MEYENBERG GOAT MILK
- Grass-fed
- High omega-3 and CLA
- No GMO
- D3 fortified
- No synthetic hormones (rBGH), antibiotics, or pesticides
- Opaque packaging

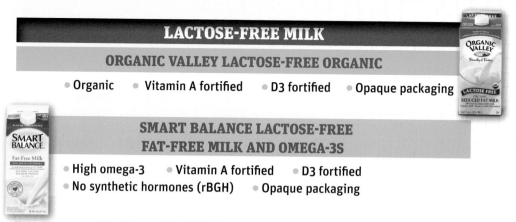

LACTOSE-FREE MILK

ORGANIC VALLEY LACTOSE-FREE ORGANIC

- Organic
- Vitamin A fortified
- D3 fortified
- Opaque packaging

SMART BALANCE LACTOSE-FREE FAT-FREE MILK AND OMEGA-3S

- High omega-3
- Vitamin A fortified
- D3 fortified
- No synthetic hormones (rBGH)
- Opaque packaging

Note: You may notice that we didn't label our organic choices as hormone (rBGH), pesticide, and antibiotic free. Remember, these facts are true of all organic products. Keep this in mind as we move through the aisles.

STEER CLEAR

MILK

HOOD CALORIE COUNTDOWN DAIRY BEVERAGE FAT FREE

When they lowered the calories in this ultra-pasteurized, non-organic milk, they added in a slew of Poor Food ingredients, including cellulose gel, cellulose gum (cheap thickener), counterfeit color, sucralose (SSS), and acesulfame potassium (SSS).

YOO HOO CHOCOLATE DRINK

We give a big Boo Hoo to this Yoo Hoo! It contains HFCS (EMD), sodium caseinate (MSG), soy lecithin and corn syrup solids (GMO), sucralose (SSS), and guar gum (EMD).

NESTLE'S COFFEE MATE CARAMEL MACCHIATO

This Coffee Mate is no mate of yours. There isn't even any dairy in this Poor Food creamer. Instead you get partially hydrogenized soybean oil (trans fat and GMO) as well as four sugary sweetener sources: corn syrup and dextrose (both GMO) and sucralose and acesulfame potassium (SSS). The nasty ingredients just keep on going.

DAIRY

- ☐ Choose unpasteurized (raw) milk.
- ☐ Choose non-homogenized milk.
- ☐ Choose milk from grass-fed cows.
- ☐ Choose organic milk.
- ☐ Choose opaque, light-blocking containers.
- ☐ Choose D3 if choosing a vitamin D fortified milk.
- ☐ Choose milk with high omega-3 content either from grass-fed cows or fortification. If fortified, we suggest a product that uses fish oil as its omega-3 source.
- ☐ Avoid flavored milks loaded with sugar and Sinister Sugar Substitutes. Remember, even organic flavored milk beverages contain sugars and are best to avoid.
- ☐ Avoid carrageenan (suspect MSG thickener).
- ☐ Avoid ultra-pasteurized dairy.

My go-to Rich Food choices for milk: _____

_____

_____

_____

_____

_____

_____

_____

_____

_____

_____

_____

RICH FOOD 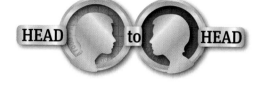 POOR FOOD

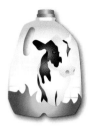

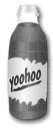

Organic, unpasteurized (raw), non-homogenized milk

Pasteurized, homogenized Yoo Hoo Chocolate Drink

150	Calories / 8 oz.	115 (2 servings per container)
Greatly increased amounts of vitamins B1, B6, B12, C, and K2, as well as calcium, phosphorous, and omega-3	Vitamins & minerals	Heating (pasteurization) destroys essential micronutrients.
300% to 500% more	CLA	Not fed grass
None permitted	Antibiotics	Common
None permitted	Synthetic Hormones	Common
GMO-free feed	GMO feed	GMO feed allowed
Nothing added GMO-free	GMO ingredients	Soy lecithin, HFCS, corn syrup solids, sodium caseinate
Lactose enzyme is intact, aiding in digestion	Lactose	Lactose enzyme is destroyed, creating allergies
All natural	Added sweeteners	HFCS, corn syrup solids, and sucralose

The raw, farm-fresh milk supplies far more micronutrients.

This milk-like drink fills you with sugars and GMOs and robs you of essential micronutrients.

DAIRY

Non-Dairy Milks

Dietary preferences or a general intolerance to dairy have led many people in search of milk alternatives. To meet the new demand, more than six hundred dairy alternatives were launched in 2010. These non-dairy milks soak, cook, blend, and strain a variety of ingredients, including soy, rice, hemp, almonds, and coconut to produce a product that, for the most part, looks and functions like real milk. Today, non-dairy milk alternatives—once packaged in shelf-stable boxes and cans, and stocked on low shelves in obscure aisles—have clamored their way into the organic and refrigerated "dairy" sections of most grocery stores. While some of these products are made with objectionable ingredients and should be avoided, many offer outstanding health benefits without the objections mentioned with dairy milk.

So, if you are in the market for a dairy alternative, we've outlined five that will help you make the Richest Food picks possible. We've ranked them from our least favorite, soy, to our top pick, coconut. While the appeal of each type of non-dairy milk may be different, there are some unwanted food additives that pop up in several different kinds of non-dairy milks. Heads up!

Soy Milk

THIS IS OUR LEAST FAVORITE in the non-dairy milk category. Let's begin with the fact that unfermented soy products, including soy milk, naturally contain two Everyday Micronutrient Depleters (high amounts of phytic acid and smaller amounts of oxalic acid).

The micronutrient-depleting effects of these EMDs aside, soy is not a recommended product for those with digestive issues, men, or young children. First, soy is not a good option for individuals with gastrointestinal conditions because it is high in oligosaccharides, a carbohydrate that is difficult for the body to break down—often causing stomach discomfort, bloating, and gas. Soy milk also contains a class of compounds called isoflavones. These compounds are classified as phytoestrogens and have been shown to mimic the effects of the female hormone estrogen in the body. Men should steer clear of isoflavones as they can cause hormone imbalances (excessive estrogen in relation to testosterone) that can lead to sexual dysfunction, reduced body hair, and even gynecomastia—the abnormal enlargement of breast tissue in males (aka "man boobs"). Additionally, parents may want to be cautious about giving their infants a soy-based formula, as some experts believe that an infant's development may be vulnerable to the estrogen-like effects of soy.

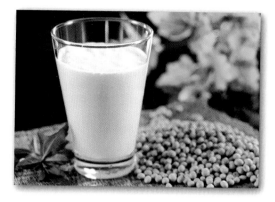

Soy milk is often heavily processed and sweetened to mask the naturally bitter taste of soybeans. If, after all this, you are still looking for a soy-based milk alternative, we suggest you choose an unsweetened, organic soy milk, as this will guarantee that you are not consuming GMO soy, which, according to the Center for Food Safety, makes up 91 percent of all soybeans on the market. It is also important to look for a product that does not contain brown rice syrup, a common soy milk sweetener, which may contain dangerously high levels of arsenic.

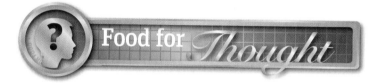

Food for *Thought*

According to *New York Times* bestselling author Ann Louise Gittleman, PhD, consuming soy milk or other soy products may cause weight gain. Soy contains goitrogens, substances that suppress the function of the thyroid gland, which can interfere with the absorption of iodine. This can cause an enlarged thyroid gland and result in weight gain—especially for the two out of three women who have borderline hypothyroidism. After just ten days without soy, Gittleman says, thyroid function should return to normal.

Rice Milk

THIS MILKY BEVERAGE, like all the milk substitutes in this category, is popular among the lactose and gluten intolerant as well as those with milk, soy, and nut allergies. However, it is high in starches and sugars and low in protein and fat, which makes it a poor choice for diabetics or those wishing to regulate carbohydrate intake. Rice milk is highly fortified because it is naturally sparse in micronutrients and may contain the EMD phytic acid if it has been made with brown rice. Additionally, recent studies have shown worrisome levels of arsenic in some rice products. (You can read more about this in Aisle 6: Grains.) Overall, rice milk is tasteless and does not typically require or contain sweeteners. This makes rice milk a slightly better option than soy milk.

Almond Milk

IF YOU'RE LACTOSE or soy intolerant and want a product containing no saturated fat or cholesterol while delivering a creamy, nutty taste, then look no further than almond milk. It is also low in calories and contains a terrific blend of micronutrients, including selenium, manganese, potassium, iron, zinc, phosphorus, calcium, vitamin E, and omega-6. But almond milk is, unfortunately, not picture perfect. Two stealth Poor Food EMDs, phytic acid and tannins, lurk within. Additionally, while omega-6 is an essential fatty acid,

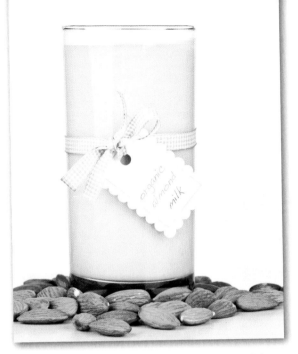

our modern too often supplies too much of it. Drinking an excess of almond milk could deliver more of the inflammation causing omega-6s than you want, especially if you are deficient in anti-inflammatory omega-3s. Finally, almond milk may not be safe for people who have nut allergies, one of the most common allergies in the United States.

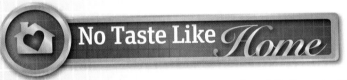

Why not improve almond milk by making it yourself with reduced EMDs and without thickeners or preservatives? Now your almond milk is All Almonds or *All*mond milk!

Homemade *All*mond Milk

DIRECTIONS

 Soak 2 cups of organic raw almonds overnight. Be sure to entirely cover almonds with water (preferably filtered) and a half tablespoon of sea salt.

 Drain off the murky water and rinse thoroughly. Blend the soaked almonds (now free of much of their phytic acid and tannins) with 4 cups of fresh water until the nuts have dissolved.

 Using a fine strainer, cheesecloth, or nut bag (yes, there are professional nut milking bags you can buy online), strain, and refrigerate.

 If desired, add a natural sweetener like stevia or an organic spice (we like 100 percent pure sugar-free vanilla) for an extra flavor kick!

Hemp Milk

ALTHOUGH HEMP MILK is made from cannabis seeds, the same as marijuana, the milk doesn't have any of the drug's psychoactive side effects. It is recommended for individuals with nut, soy, and lactose allergies who are looking for a product that contains both omega-3 and omega-6 fatty acids. Hemp milk has a 3-to-1 ratio of omega-6 to omega-3. While this ratio falls within the recommended guidelines of most nutritionists, we recommend that you strive to achieve a ratio closer to 1 to 1. The Standard American Diet can deliver a pro-inflammatory omega-6:omega-3 ratio of 20 to 1 or worse. It should be noted that the omega-3 in hemp is ALA, the only form of omega-3 found in plants, and doesn't have all the great benefits of omega-3 fish oils, which naturally contain the other two forms of omega-3, EPA and DHA.

Unlike the other milk stand-ins discussed thus far, hemp is not thought to contain any of the EMDs (phytic acid, oxalic acid, or tannins) and is an excellent source of magnesium, which puts hemp near our top pick. Both original and flavored hemp beverages are often loaded with sweeteners and thickening agents, so read labels carefully and try to find organic brands from reputable companies.

Coconut Milk

PERHAPS THE SWEETEST and creamiest option in the non-dairy milk category—and our personal favorite—is coconut milk. Coconut milk naturally boosts the immune system by means of its great micronutrient content (including calcium, magnesium, potassium, phosphorus, manganese, copper, zinc, iron, selenium, and vitamins C and E). The manganese in coconut is great for diabetics, while the potassium in coconut milk can aid in lowering blood pressure. This milk alternative contains a type of fat known as MCT (medium-chain triglycerides), which are anti-viral and anti-bacterial. What's more, MCTs are converted almost immediately into energy, so they are less likely to be stored as body fat and can actually assist in the metabolism of stored fat. So many great benefits—which is why we are cuckoo for coconuts!

As with the other milk alternatives, all of the refrigerated coconut beverage companies sneak in sugars, preservatives, and thickeners. There are better, more additive-free products in the shelf-stable area, but not all of them use BPA-free packaging, so beware.

DAIRY

STEER HERE

SOY MILK

WHOLE FOODS BRAND 365 ORGANIC SOY MILK

- Organic
- Sweetener free
- Still contains carrageenan

RICE MILK

SHELF STABLE ORGANIC RICE DREAM ENRICHED ORIGINAL

- Organic
- Sweetener free

WEGMANS ORGANIC ORIGINAL RICE BEVERAGE

- Organic
- Sweetener free

ALMOND MILK

HOMEMADE *ALLMOND* MILK

- Organic
- Sweetener free

WHOLE FOODS 365 EVERYDAY VALUE ORGANIC ALMOND MILK UNSWEETENED

- Organic
- The source of vitamin E is synthetic, dl-alpha-tocopherol acetate
- Carrageenan is swapped for less-offensive xantham gum

BLUE DIAMOND ALMOND, ALMOND BREEZE UNSWEETENED ORIGINAL

- Sweetener free
- Still contains carrageenan
- A stand out for adding the natural source, d-alpha-tocopherol, for vitamin E

HEMP MILK

LIVING HARVEST TEMPT UNSWEETENED CREAMY NON-DAIRY VANILLA (OR ORIGINAL) HEMPMILK BEVERAGE

- Sweetener free
- Still contains carrageenan

COCONUT MILK

NATURAL VALUE ORGANIC COCONUT MILK

- BPA-free can
- Sweetener free
- Thickener free

TRADER JOE'S LIGHT COCONUT MILK

- BPA-free can
- Sweetener free
- Thickener free

AROY–D 100% COCONUT MILK ORIGINAL

- BPA-free cartons
- Sweetener free
- Thickener free

STEER CLEAR

MILK ALTERNATIVES

SILK SOYMILK CHOCOLATE

We applaud Silk products for using non-GMO soy. However, this soy is not organic, so it can still be a source of pesticides and unhealthy fertilizers. It also contains carrageenan (MSG), and has 200 percent more sugar (EMD), in the form of "all natural" evaporated cane juice, than the Silk Soymilk Original.

SHOPRITE ORGANIC RICE MILK VANILLA

Don't be fooled by the word *organic*. One look at the ingredients, and you will notice there is no rice in this product at all! Instead, it is made with brown rice syrup, which not only may contain arsenic but also intensely spikes insulin, scoring an 85 on the glycemic index.

ALMOND BREEZE VANILLA ALMOND MILK

It's a breeze to spot the Poor Food ingredients in this product. On top of adding evaporated cane juice, aka sugar (EMD), as its second-listed ingredient, this product adds carrageenan (MSG) and non-organic soy lecithin (most likely GMO soy) to the carton.

LIVING HARVEST TEMPT CREAMY NON-DAIRY BEVERAGE VANILLA

Don't be tempted to put this in your cart. Two of the three top ingredients in this carrageenan-thickened beverage are unwanted sweeteners (evaporated cane juice and brown rice syrup).

ROLAND CLASSIC COCONUT MILK

This Classic Poor Food contains guar gum (EMD) and sulfites (EMD) that most canned coconut milks leave out and is packaged in BPA cans.

DAIRY

- ☐ **Choose organic.**
- ☐ **Choose BPA-free cartons and cans.**
- ☐ Avoid carrageenan, guar gum, and pectin.
- ☐ Avoid HFCS, evaporated cane juice, dextrose, brown rice syrup, and sugar.
- ☐ Avoid artificial flavors.

*My go-to Rich Food choices for dairy products:*_____

_____

_____

_____

_____

_____

_____

_____

_____

_____

_____

_____

_____

_____

_____

_____

_____

_____

_____

Yogurt, Greek Yogurt, and Kefir

Can you guess the single food that has been shown to have the strongest link to long-term weight loss? That's right—yogurt! In a 2011 study published in the *New England Journal of Medicine,* 120,000 adults were followed for two decades. Those who ate one cup of yogurt daily spooned their way thin. Whether your preference is good old-fashioned yogurt, the chic Greek yogurt, or kefir, a unique yogurt-like drink, the added dietary calcium and phosphorous contained in all three can strengthen tooth enamel, prevent cavities, and reduce the risk of osteoporosis. However, while these dairy delights may offer similar micronutrient benefits, the probiotic benefits can be greatly different.

You hear a lot about the beneficial probiotics in yogurt, but it may surprise you that not all store-bought brands deliver on these promises. All yogurts are made by first adding two types of bacteria to milk, *lactobacillus bulgaricus* and *streptococcus thermophilus.* Collectively, these bacteria are known as acidophilus. The yogurts are then heated, which is when yogurt can take two different nutritional paths. You see, the process of heating the yogurt actually kills off those beneficial bacteria, and only *some* manufacturers add more in at this late stage to make the treat full of tummy-taming cultures. It is these newly added beneficial bacteria, those that are still *live* and *active,* that keep your digestive system clean.

According to researchers from the Jean Mayer USDA Human Nutrition Research Center on Aging at Tufts University, the live active cultures may help prevent certain gastrointestinal conditions, including lactose intolerance, constipation, diarrhea, colon cancer, inflammatory bowel disease (IBD), and H. pylori infections. Additionally, these live active probiotic bacteria in yogurt and kefir can rev up your immune system by increasing the production of the infection-fighting protein *interferon-gamma* by 400 percent. This can reduce your risk of yeast infections, prevent allergy symptoms, and naturally increase your metabolism.

However, read labels carefully. Remember, while all yogurts are made with those two strands of live cultures, many don't survive the heat treatments. Don't let the manufacturers fool you with "made with live active cultures," or by putting them in the ingredient list. They may have started out there, but you can only be sure they survived by checking the labels for the words "*contains* active cultures, *active* yogurt cultures, or *living* yogurt cultures." Many larger companies actually perform testing and proudly display the National Yogurt Association's LAC (Live Active Cultures) seal.

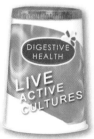

Greek yogurt is made by triple straining yogurt to remove greater amounts of the watery whey. This creates a thick, rich product with almost twice the protein and half the carbohydrates and sodium of regular yogurt. In fact, one small container of Greek yogurt packs the same amount of protein as a can of tuna! Many people prefer the taste and texture of Greek yogurt and often compare it to ice cream.

Last, kefir, meaning "good feeling" in Turkish, is a thin yogurt-like drink that is made by adding kefir grains (not real grains, but a symbiotic combination of bacteria and yeast that looks like cauliflower) to cow, sheep, goat, or camel milk (cow milk is used in the United States), which produces a slightly fizzy, sour-tasting drink. Kefir is a mainstay in the Middle East and Eastern Europe and has gained popularity in recent years in the United States for its probiotic benefits. Research shows that kefir has even more beneficial bacteria than yogurt and a higher nutritional value because it is made with bacteria and yeast.

When Good Yogurts Go Bad

AS WITH THE MILK DISCUSSED EARLIER, our Rich Food choices are not based on whether your yogurt or kefir is made from full-fat or low-fat milk. Your personal dietary profile will dictate whether you look to higher fat or lower fat products. What we want you to remember is that most of the time when the fat comes out, something else must go in to take its place. Food scientists have invented all sorts of thickeners and additives to help make low-fat products look and taste as thick and delicious as their full-fat counterparts. Make sure you read the ingredients carefully to avoid these additives.

We are also not fans of yogurt and kefir that resemble sugary fruit-flavored desserts rather than the wholesome, micronutrient- and bacteria-rich foods they are meant to be. Yes, adding fresh berries, nuts or seeds, and assorted fruits is a delicious and nutritious way to add personality to your morning bowl of yogurt, but why should yogurt and kefir taste like cherry cheesecake, key lime pie, strawberry lemonade, or margaritas? To create these artificial flavors, manufacturers must add in a slew of Poor Food ingredients, including assorted forms of sugar, thickening agents, and artificial colors.

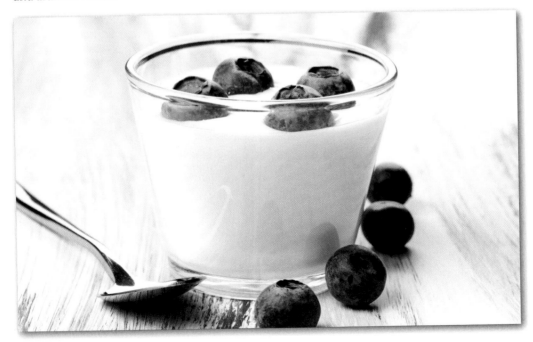

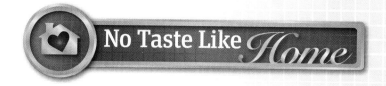

Why not get all the health benefits of raw, unpasteurized, non-homogenized milk in yogurt as well? Yogurt was discovered accidentally in primitive times when milk was stored in warm climates. So, recreating a warm climate can change your milk into delicious yogurt. Our simple recipe consists of micronutrient-rich ingredients and can be made while you are at work or sound sleep.

Yummy Tummy Yogurt

WHAT YOU WILL NEED
- 4 quart-size glass canning jars with lids
- Thermometer
- Large pot. Use a pot that is at least 1 ½ gallons so the milk doesn't crawl up as it heats.
- Oven
- Dutch oven
- Towels

INGREDIENTS
- 1 gallon milk (preferably unpasteurized, full-fat for creamier, thicker yogurt)
- 1 cup yogurt starter (you can use a cup from your last batch of homemade yogurt or from an unflavored store-bought brand that has live, active cultures)

DIRECTIONS

 1 In large pot, heat milk to just below boiling, 200 degrees Fahrenheit. Stir milk gently as it heats to make sure it doesn't boil over or scorch bottom of pan.

 2 Let milk cool to 112 to 115 degrees Fahrenheit. To hurry process, place pan in ice water. Gently stir milk as it cools.

 3 Pour about a cup of the warmed milk into small bowl and whisk in the yogurt starter. Once dissolved, whisk the mixture into the pot of remaining warmed milk.

 4 Pour mixture into the four glass jars and cover. If you don't have a yogurt-making machine that stabilizes the temperature for you, simply warm your oven to 115 degrees Fahrenheit. Then wrap the four sealed glass jars with towels to keep them warm and snug. Place the wrapped jars in a Dutch oven and cover with lid.

 5 Turn off oven and close.

 6 Be patient for about six hours. The longer the yogurt incubates, the richer the yogurt.

 7 Refrigerate and enjoy!

If you love homemade yogurt, like we do, you may want to purchase a yogurt maker. This eliminates the need for the oven incubation with towels and Dutch oven and makes yogurt making a snap. You can find our product suggestion in our Real Food Resource Center online at CaltonNutrition.com/Rich-food-marketplace.aspx.

DAIRY

STEER HERE

YOGURT

OUR TOP PICK! Homemade yogurt (Yummy Tummy Yogurt) or kefir made from grass-fed, unpasteurized, non-homogenized milk or cream.

TRADERS POINT CREAMERY PLAIN YOGURT

- Organic
- Grass-fed
- Non-homogenized
- Live active cultures
- High omega-3s and CLA

KALONA SUPERNATURAL ORGANIC WHOLE MILK PLAIN YOGURT

- Organic
- Non-homogenized
- Live active cultures

TRADER JOE'S EUROPEAN STYLE THICK & CREAMY ORGANIC PLAIN NONFAT YOGURT

- Organic
- Live active cultures

GREEK YOGURT

TRADERS POINT CREAMERY GREEK YOGURT

- Organic
- Grass-fed
- Non-homogenized
- Live active cultures
- High omega-3s and CLA

NANCY'S ORGANIC WHOLE MILK PLAIN PROBIOTIC GREEK YOGURT

- Organic
- Live active cultures

STONYFIELD GREEK YOGURT

- Organic
- Live active cultures
- Now available in non-fat and low-fat versions

This product was previously Stonyfield Oikos, but they recently changed the name.

KEFIR

LIFEWAY ORGANIC WHOLE AND LOW-FAT, PLAIN UNSWEETENED KEFIR

- Organic
- Grass-fed
- Live active cultures
- High omega-3s and CLA

GREEN VALLEY LACTOSE FREE ORGANIC PLAIN KEFIR

- Organic
- Grass-fed
- Live active cultures
- High omega-3s and CLA

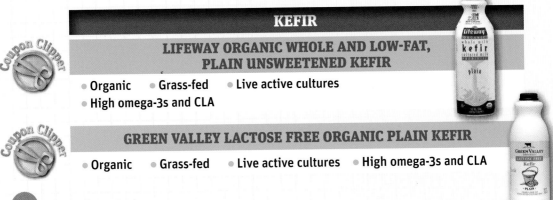

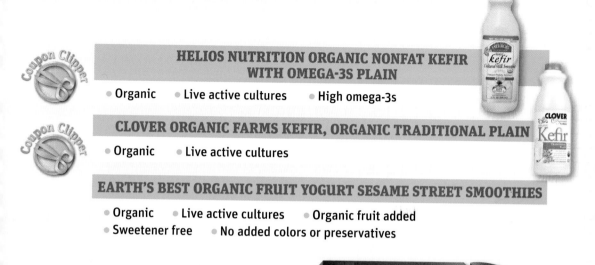

Coupon Clipper

Coupon Clipper

HELIOS NUTRITION ORGANIC NONFAT KEFIR WITH OMEGA-3S PLAIN

- Organic
- Live active cultures
- High omega-3s

CLOVER ORGANIC FARMS KEFIR, ORGANIC TRADITIONAL PLAIN

- Organic
- Live active cultures

EARTH'S BEST ORGANIC FRUIT YOGURT SESAME STREET SMOOTHIES

- Organic
- Live active cultures
- Organic fruit added
- Sweetener free
- No added colors or preservatives

STEER CLEAR

YOGURT, GREEK YOGURT, AND KEFIR

WEIGHT WATCHERS BLACK CHERRY

Watch out for this one! This non-organic option cons you with counterfeit colors (blue #1 is illegal in other countries, and red #40 may be carcinogenic), and tricks your taste buds with added sucralose (Sinister Sugar Substitute) and crystalline fructose (a GMO sweetener). Formulated to enhance your diet, this creamy concoction contains gelatin, an irreversibly hydrolyzed form of collagen. Did you catch the word *hydrolyzed?* That's right—MSG, which has been cause to induce weight gain, has been added into this diet disaster.

YOPLAIT LIGHT FAT-FREE RASPBERRY LEMONADE

There is nothing refreshing about these yogurt ingredients. While rBGH free, this yogurt contains HFCS (EMD), modified cornstarch (GMO), aspartame (SSS), and artificial color red #40 (counterfeit color).

YOCRUNCH GREEK YOGURT PEACH WITH GRANOLA

This non-organic Greek yogurt contains sugar, maltodextrin, modified food starch, more sugar, soluble corn fiber, wheat, rice, molasses, canola oil, and soy lecithin. It is time to throw away this EMD and GMO filled Yo' mess!

LIFEWAY NONFAT STRAWBERRY GREEK STYLE KEFIR

Step away from this particular Lifeway Kefir. It contains evaporated cane juice (sugar), strawberry juice concentrate (sugar), and potential pesticide and GMO exposure. There is more sugar here than in a package of Twix Caramel Cookie Bars.

DAIRY

GoHurt is more like it! These addictive, sugary messes each contain the equivalent to five packets of sugar. Leave them on store shelves and save your children from the sugar, HFCS, artificial colors (linked with ADHD), and GMO ingredients.

☐ Choose homemade yogurts or kefirs from unpasteurized milk.

☐ Choose a product that contains live active cultures.

☐ Choose grass-fed and organic options.

☐ Choose yogurts with minimal ingredients.

☐ Avoid all forms of added sugars.

☐ Avoid starches and thickeners.

☐ Avoid artificial colors and flavors.

☐ Avoid products with added granolas, candy, and fruit mix-ins.

☐ Remember that some companies that are not organic still use dairy that is rBGH/rBST and antibiotic free.

My go-to Rich Food choices for yogurt, greek yogurt, and kefir: _____

_____

_____

_____

_____

_____

_____

_____

_____

_____

_____

Sour Cream

Taco night and loaded baked potatoes would seem naked without this deliciously rich dairy topping. But what exactly is sour cream, and how is it made? Traditionally, cream is soured by adding lactic acid bacteria, which naturally thickens and sours the dairy, creating a topping that is filled with probiotics that aid in digestion. Unfortunately, today, the desire to maximize profits, as well as to create low-fat and non-fat alternatives, has brought us far from this traditional practice. Many of today's products contain no cream or live cultures and are loaded with modified cornstarch, thickeners, and flavoring agents. In fact, some sour creams even add in artificial colors to make the white cream appear whiter.

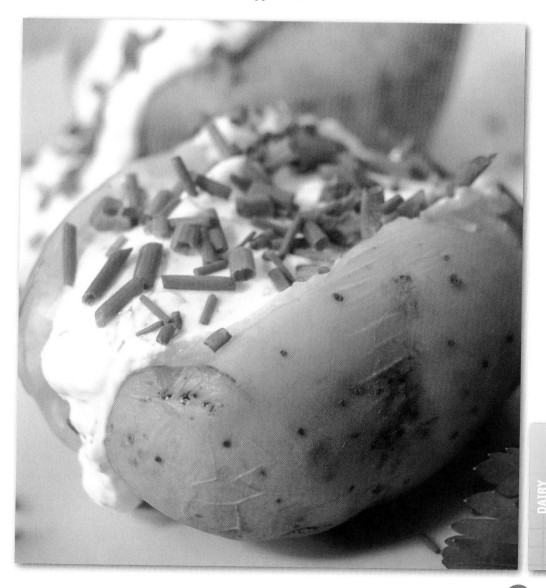

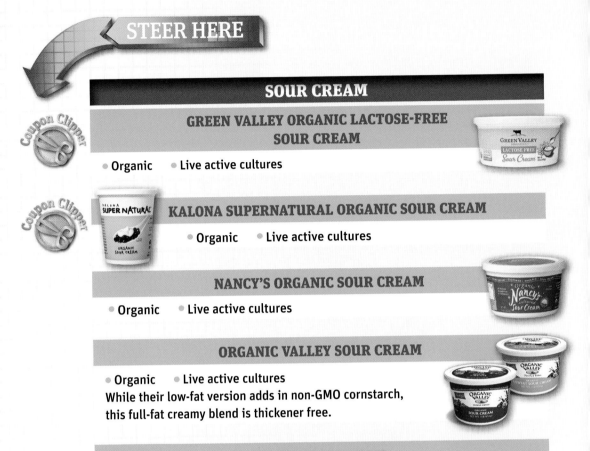

STEER HERE

SOUR CREAM

GREEN VALLEY ORGANIC LACTOSE-FREE SOUR CREAM

- Organic
- Live active cultures

KALONA SUPERNATURAL ORGANIC SOUR CREAM

- Organic
- Live active cultures

NANCY'S ORGANIC SOUR CREAM

- Organic
- Live active cultures

ORGANIC VALLEY SOUR CREAM

- Organic
- Live active cultures

While their low-fat version adds in non-GMO cornstarch, this full-fat creamy blend is thickener free.

DAISY SOUR CREAM

- Live active cultures
- No synthetic hormones
- Best of the brands in conventional supermarkets

CABOT SOUR CREAM

Start with sad steer that have been fed GMO-laden grain feed and treated with hormones while living on a factory farm. Add in modified cornstarch (GMO), carrageenan (MSG) and guar gum (EMD), and you have a recipe for a Poor Food.

BREAKSTONE'S FAT FREE SOUR CREAM

First of all, the name is sour *cream,* so we know that any fat-free version must be a chemistry experiment in disguise. A dollop of this disaster places dried corn syrup (sugary GMO), modified food starch (GMO), maltodextrin (GMO sugar), xanthan gum, and natural flavor (we suspect MSG) in your dish. Breakstone's also sneaks in artificial colors to whiten and brighten!

TOFUTTI SOUR SUPREME

While Tofutti says they never use GMO soy protein and get all other soy derivatives from non-GMO sources when available, we still give it thumbs down for the Poor Food ingredients in this "science cream," including hydrogenated soybean oil (trans fat), mono and diglycerides (more trans fats), isolated soy protein (the word *protein* should remind you it is a source of MSG), maltodextrin (sugar), tofu (more goitrogenic soy), sugar (EMD), and carrageenan and guar gum (adding possible MSG, EMD, and stomach upset).

Cottage Cheese

Popular with dieters, these chunky cheese curds suffer from many of the same problems as the previous dairy delights.

STEER HERE

COTTAGE CHEESE

TRADERS POINT CREAMERY COTTAGE CHEESE

- Organic
- Grass-fed
- Non-homogenized
- Live active cultures
- High omega-3 and CLA

NANCY ORGANIC LOW FAT COTTAGE CHEESE

- Organic
- Live active cultures

KALONA SUPERNATURAL REGULAR AND REDUCED FAT ORGANIC COTTAGE CHEESES

- Organic
- Non-homogenized
- Live active cultures
- Uses unrefined Celtic sea salt—bonus!

DAISY COTTAGE CHEESE & LOW FAT COTTAGE CHEESE

- No synthetic hormones
- Best of the brands in conventional supermarkets

HORIZON ORGANIC COTTAGE CHEESE

- Organic
- Live active cultures
- Still contains carrageenan
- Fortified with 200 percent more bone-building calcium

Coupon Clipper

WALMART BRAND GREAT VALUE COTTAGE CHEESE

We don't care how much we save—putting in all of these ingredients is a very poor choice even if Walmart is using hormone-free dairy: maltodextrin (GMO sugar), phosphoric acid (EMD), guar gum (EMD), carrageenan (MSG), modified cornstarch (GMO), and dextrose (more sugar).

BREAKSTONE'S COTTAGE DOUBLE 100 CALORIE WITH PINEAPPLE

This 100-calorie snack has nearly as much sugar as two fun-size Snickers bars. This non-organic dairy is filled with HFCS (EMD/GMO), sugar (EMD), and modified food starch (GMO).

- ☐ Choose organic.
- ☐ Choose non-homogenized.
- ☐ Choose foods that *contain* "living" or "active" cultures.
- ☐ Avoid sweeteners, thickeners, and GMO ingredients.
- ☐ Avoid cottage cheese with fruit mix-ins.

*My go-to Rich Food choices for sour cream and cottage cheese:*_____

_____

_____

_____

_____

_____

_____

_____

Checkout Checklist

DAIRY

RICH FOOD vs. POOR FOOD

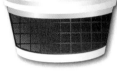

HEAD to HEAD

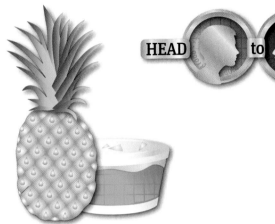

Nancy's Organic Low Fat Cottage Cheese with fresh pineapple

Breakstone's Cottage Double with pineapple

100 75 from cottage cheese 25 from pineapple	Calories	100
.9 g	Fat	1.5 g
7.8 g	Sugar	14 g
13.5 g	Protein	8 g
None permitted	Hormones	rBGH and rBST allowed
GMO-free feed	GMO feed	GMO feed allowed
Nothing added; GMO free	GMO ingredients	Cornstarch and HFCS
All natural	Added sweeteners	HFCS and sugar
Live cultures for healthy gut	Healthy Bacteria	None here

The healthy gut bacteria in Rich Food cottage cheeses can aid in digestion, reduce bloating, and maximize weight loss.

Fewer micronutrients and active cultures with more hormones, GMOs, and sugars to spike insulin and fat storage.

Cheese

Depending on who you listen to, there are between four hundred and one thousand different varieties of cheese! While all cheese starts off in block form, grocery stores are filled with sliced, shredded, grated, and crumbled options. While they may be convenient, they may not be your best choice from a nutritional perspective.

To begin with, as cheese is sliced, shredded, grated, and crumbled into smaller pieces with more surface area, greater amounts of the product become exposed to light and air (both EMDs). In addition, while we would expect cheese slices to be pre-sliced versions of block cheeses, many add in an ingredient known as natamycin, an antibiotic-based mold inhibitor. While it is considered safe in small doses, this medicinal add-in is fairly new, and we prefer it be left out. As we further diminish the cheese sizes to those shredded, grated, and crumbled products, manufacturers add in anticaking agents such as potato starch, calcium sulphate (or similar), and cellulose powder.

Not familiar with cellulose powder? Well, this ingredient found in nearly every shredded cheese on the market is really wood pulp, which contains an indigestible fiber that absorbs moisture in packaging to extend the food's shelf life inexpensively. Ask yourself if you would still buy the shredded cheese if the packaging advertised, *"Shredded cheddar and tree bark."* Our suggestion is to buy your cheese the way it was traditionally made, as a block. Then, cut, shred, or crumble it yourself right before you are going to eat it. This maximizes micronutrient values and protects you from the aforementioned objectionable additives.

Also, spend some time in the artisan cheese section of

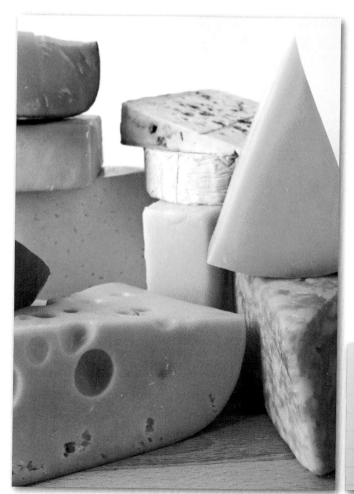

your supermarket. You know—the spot where they sell the fancy cheeses, not the pre-sliced cheddar and provolone. Did you know that many of these areas stock a large assortment of rBGH-free cheeses? You may not, because many of them aren't labeled as such. You should also know that all cheese that comes from Canada or the European Union is automatically rBGH free, due to their ban on this hormone. Don't forget the importance of grass-fed cheese, either—cows fed their naturally preferred feed (grass) produce cheese up to 400 times richer in fat-metabolizing CLA. And because all cheese was once milk, and we know that raw milk is the most micronutrient rich, we should be on the lookout for raw cheeses. Unlike raw milk, which most often cannot be found in the grocery store, raw cheeses are quite common. Many blue cheeses and European cheeses are made with raw milk.

Wondering how your freshly sliced deli cheeses stack up? Most of these cheeses are not organic or grass-fed, and because they have been manufactured in the United States, the majority of them will have been made from cows treated with rBGH. Even trusted brands like Boars Head still use hormone-tainted milk in their deli slices. While the antibiotic natamycin has been eliminated in the deli options, we wouldn't suggest these cheeses as our grocery store picks. However, if you still love the convenience of deli sliced cheeses, search for those labeled as organic or imported.

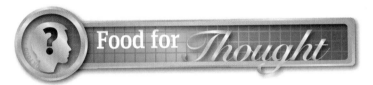

Here is some goooda news about Gouda (wow, that was cheesy!). This cheese of Dutch origin is the third-highest source of the elusive vitamin K2, supplying nearly 100 percent of your daily requirement (RDI) in a mere 3.5-ounce serving. Only *natto*, a Japanese fermented soybean dish, and goose liver paté surpass it. There are two natural forms of vitamin K: K1, which comes from plants and is essential for blood clotting, and K2, which comes from bacterial/animal sources and may reduce the risk of osteoporosis, arterial calcification, rheumatoid arthritis, and even certain types of cancer.

While many people take in a lot of dietary K1 through green vegetables, K1 is thought to convert into K2 at only a rate of approximately 10 to 1, which doesn't afford us much access to all the incredible health benefits of K2. Even the individuals eating K2-rich animal sources on a regular basis, like grass-fed meats and dairy products and pastured eggs, may find it difficult to be sufficient in this essential fat-soluble vitamin. Gouda to the rescue! This mild, nutty, creamy cheese is an easy, inexpensive, and delicious way to ingest K2. Oh, and Gouda is high in K2 even if it is not from a grass-fed or raw source, because the majority of the K2 comes from the bacterial cultures used to ferment the milk into Gouda. Grab a block of it today!

STEER HERE

OUR TOP PICK! Organic, raw cheeses from grass-fed cows

BLOCK CHEESE

U.S. WELLNESS MEATS ORGANIC RAW CHEESE (THREE VARIETIES)

- Unpasteurized
- Organic
- Grass-fed
- High omega-3s and CLA

RUMIANO FAMILY ORGANIC CHEESE (ALL VARIETIES)

- Organic
- Grass-fed
- High omega-3s and CLA

Don't miss their incredible sliced options as well.

ORGANIC VALLEY RAW CHEESE (ALL VARIETIES)

- Unpasteurized
- Organic

KERRYGOLD CHEESE (ALL VARIETIES)

- No synthetic hormones (rBGH free)
- Grass-fed
- High omega-3s and CLA

Kerrygold discloses "that approximately 3 percent of a cow's total typical annual diet may be from GM sources."

TRADER JOE'S RAW MILK CHEDDAR CHEESE

- Unpasteurized

SLICED CHEESE

ORGANIC VALLEY AMERICAN SINGLES

- Organic
- Anticaking additive free

APPLEGATE FARMS CHEESES (ALL VARIETIES)

- Organic
- Anticaking additive free

APPLEGATE FARMS YOGURT CHEESE

- Live active cultures
- No synthetic hormones (rBGH free)
- Lactose Free
- Anticaking additive free

HORIZON ORGANIC CHEDDAR CHEESE SLICES

- Organic
- Anticaking additive free

SHREDDED CHEESE

Sorry, no luck in the shredded cheese department. All of the in-store, pre-shredded products add in far too much cellulose and anticaking ingredients. Time to buy a cheese grater.

CRUMBLED CHEESE

ORGANIC VALLEY BLUE CHEESE CRUMBLES

- Organic
- Anticaking additive free

SPREADABLE CHEESE

FAYETTE CREAMERY CHEESE COLD PACK, HORSERADISH RAW MILK CHEDDAR

- Unpasteurized

CREAM CHEESE

NANCY'S ORGANIC CULTURED CREAM CHEESE

- Organic
- Non-homogenized whole cream

RICOTTA CHEESE

NATURAL BY NATURE RICOTTA

- Organic
- Grass-fed
- High omega-3s and CLA

ORGANIC VALLEY WHOLE MILK RICOTTA

- Organic

WEGMANS BRAND

- Not organic, but leaves out the thickeners
- No synthetic hormones (rBGH free)

STEER CLEAR

BLOCK CHEESE

KAUKAUNA PORT WINE BALL, COLD PACK WITH ALMONDS

You'll start bawling when you read the label. Although not sliced or shredded, this cheese contains partially hydrogenated corn oil (trans fat, GMO), liquid corn oil (GMO), guar gum (EMD), and blue #2 and red #40.

SLICED CHEESE

KRAFT SINGLES FAT FREE AMERICAN

Keep your kids away from these non-organic (Kraft still uses rBGH) American singles if you want to avoid hormones, antibiotics, GMOs, pesticides, dried corn syrup (EMD, GMO), artificial color (CC), carrageenan (MSG), cellulose gum (wood pulp), artificial flavor (why does cheese need flavor?), and disodium inosinate (MSG indicator).

SHREDDED CHEESE

CRACKER BARREL SHREDS ALL TYPES

Not all cheeses are as good as they are cracked up to be. This shredded cheese is not organic or rBGH-free and contains the trifecta of anticaking additives (potato starch, powdered cellulose, and calcium sulphate) as well as natamycin.

SPREADABLE CHEESE

KRAFT CHEEZ WHIZ SQUEEZE AND KRAFT EASY CHEESE

These two cheezes tie for our Steer Clear choice in the spreadable cheese category. Just in case you are tempted by these canned and bottled catastrophes, here are a few of their Poor Food ingredients: dried corn syrup, modified food starch, corn syrup, caramel color, sugar, hydrolyzed corn protein, monosodium glutamate, and artificial colors.

CREAM CHEESE

MY ESSENTIALS FAT FREE CREAM CHEESE

This is what happens when you try to make a fat-free cream cheese. The Poor Food ingredients include sugar, artificial color, guar gum, carrageenan, corn syrup solids, and modified food starch, all of which have an asterisk, which states, "ingredient not in regular cream cheese." The guar gum and carrageenan have a double asterisk stating that "ingredients are in excess of amount allowed in regular cream cheese."

DAIRY

LIFEWAY SWEET KISS CHEESE SPREAD CHOCOLATE CHIP

A perfect example of a good cream cheese gone very wrong. This sweet kiss comes with three different sources of sugar, partially hydrogenated soybean oil, cornstarch, artificial flavors, soy lecithin, and dextrose.

RICOTTA CHEESE

POLLY-O RICOTTA

O-My God, this ricotta is packed with Poor Food ingredients. This non-organic dairy is filled with growth hormones and a trifecta of MSG and EMD thickeners (carrageenan, guar gum, and xanthan gum).

☐ Choose organic cheese.

☐ Choose unpasteurized cheese generally labeled as raw cheese.

☐ Choose grass-fed cheese.

☐ If not choosing organic cheese, choose cheese made from rBGH/rBST-free dairy cows. Purchasing cheeses made in Europe or Canada guarantees this.

☐ Choose block cheese, and cut, chop, and shred yourself.

☐ Avoid cellulose, natamycin, potato starch, calcium sulphate, and any other additives labeled as anticaking or antimicrobial.

☐ Avoid MSG and EMD thickeners.

My go-to Rich Food choices for cheese: _____

_____

_____

_____

_____

Butter

Butter is churned cream, so everything you have already learned concerning the benefits of organic, grass-fed, unpasteurized milk applies to butter. Grass-fed butter has higher quantities of the essential micronutrients, and grass-fed dairy cows produce butter that has 50 percent more of the vitamins E and A and nearly 400 percent more beta-carotene (which gives the grass-fed butter its deeper yellow color) than the butter produced from factory-farmed cows.

While beta-carotene is naturally occurring in butter, you may see it as an ingredient in some butter alternatives. These margarines and vegetable oils use the vitamin's natural orange pigment to transform their often waxy, shortening-like spreads and sprays into something more appealing and familiar. You also want to consider what type of oil is being used. Many of the products in years past were filled with hydrogenated vegetable oils—those man-made trans fats that have been shown to increase the risk of coronary heart disease and have been outlawed in restaurants in numerous large US cities, thanks to a charge led by New York City beginning back in 2005. While many products have reduced the trans fats, the types and sources of the oils themselves are still troublesome because they mostly come from genetically modified corn and soybean oils. (For more information on these man-made oils, turn to Aisle 7: Baking.) Luckily, there are some new superstars in the bevy of butter options. While we opt for raw, grass-fed butter in our home, we have chosen our top picks here for you, whether you want butter, light butter, or a butter alternative.

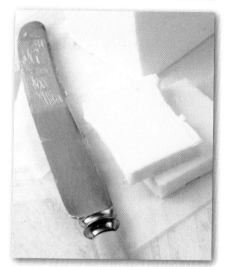

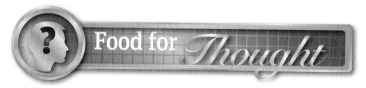

Is organic butter really that much better? You butter believe it! We've shared with you the dangers of bovine growth hormones (rBGH/rBST) and explained that organic milk guarantees you will not be ingesting these carcinogens. However, we want to stress that it is even more important to buy organic butter, because these same unwanted hormones actually accumulate in the highest concentration in butterfat. So, drinking hormone-infused milk is one thing, but eating butter churned from that milk really increases your exposure. You'll *never* encounter or consume these contaminants if you always remember to buy organic butter.

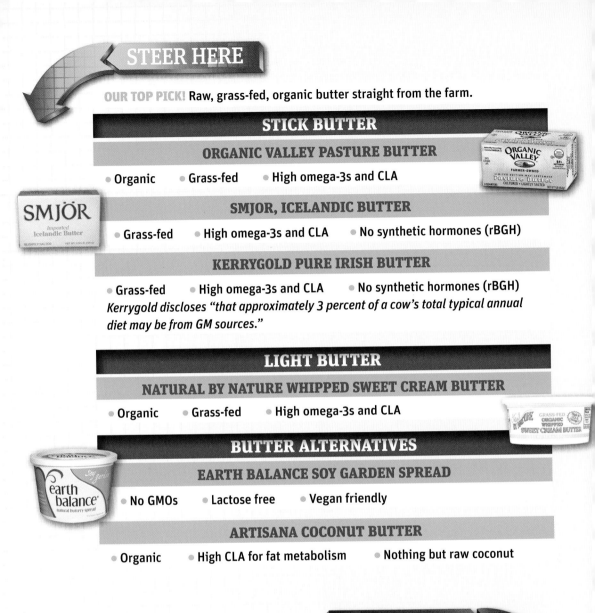

STEER HERE

OUR TOP PICK! Raw, grass-fed, organic butter straight from the farm.

STICK BUTTER

ORGANIC VALLEY PASTURE BUTTER

- Organic
- Grass-fed
- High omega-3s and CLA

SMJOR, ICELANDIC BUTTER

- Grass-fed
- High omega-3s and CLA
- No synthetic hormones (rBGH)

KERRYGOLD PURE IRISH BUTTER

- Grass-fed
- High omega-3s and CLA
- No synthetic hormones (rBGH)

Kerrygold discloses "that approximately 3 percent of a cow's total typical annual diet may be from GM sources."

LIGHT BUTTER

NATURAL BY NATURE WHIPPED SWEET CREAM BUTTER

- Organic
- Grass-fed
- High omega-3s and CLA

BUTTER ALTERNATIVES

EARTH BALANCE SOY GARDEN SPREAD

- No GMOs
- Lactose free
- Vegan friendly

ARTISANA COCONUT BUTTER

- Organic
- High CLA for fat metabolism
- Nothing but raw coconut

STEER CLEAR

STICK BUTTER

LAND O' LAKES MARGARINE 80% VEGETABLE OIL

Don't be fooled using this butter bomb on your vegetables. It has the highest trans fat content of any stick butter/margarine we found. With 2.5 grams of trans fat from partially hydrogenated soybean oil (GMO) and liquid soybean oil (GMO), soy lecithin (GMO), and artificial flavor, you should easily be able to identify this stick as a Poor Food.

LIGHT BUTTER

SHEDD'S SPREAD COUNTRY CROCK HONEY SPREAD

Everything butter should not be, in our opinion. When you put this sweet spread on your food, you are adding liquid soybean oil (GMO), partially hydrogenated soybean oil (trans fat and GMO), high fructose corn syrup (GMO, EMD), calcium disodium EDTA (EMD), and artificial flavors.

BUTTER ALTERNATIVES

I CAN'T BELIEVE IT'S NOT BUTTER SPRAY

After scrutinizing the ingredients, we certainly can believe it's not butter. According to the Nutrition Facts, this 12-ounce bottle contains 1,700 servings (Really?) Who are they trying to fool? That means if you use one serving per day, this bottle would last you more than four-and-a-half years. And just in case you were wondering how it was that a product made out of pure fat (soybean oil/GMO), emulsifiers (soy lecithin/GMO), preservatives (sodium benzoate/allergen and calcium disodium EDTA/EMD), and flavors (includes artificial flavors) can have zero calories and zero fat, we are here to tell you it doesn't!

According to the FDA Food Labeling Guide, a product can claim zero calories and zero fat if a serving contains less that 5 calories and .5 grams of fat. That means that based on the likelihood that each serving has the most amount of fat legally allowed (.49 gm), we can calculate that the grams of fat in the 12-ounce bottle are close to (1,700 x .49 = 833) 833 grams. When we multiply that by 9 (the calories in 1 gram of fat), we can see that the 12-ounce bottle contains approximately 7,497 calories. That's more calories and fat than *four* 8-ounce Rich Food Organic Valley Pasture butter blocks—not really a low calorie/fat alternative at all.

☐ Choose raw (unpasteurized) butter.

☐ Choose grass-fed butter.

☐ Choose organic butter.

☐ Choose butter from dairy cows that do not receive rBGH. (All Canadian and European butters do not contain this.)

☐ Avoid GMO oil products masquerading as butter.

☐ Avoid sprays and squeeze containers of butter.

☐ Avoid trans fats in stick margarines.

My go-to Rich Food choices for butter: _____

Checkout Checklist

DAIRY

Eggs

We realize that eggs are not technically dairy products because they aren't bred from Bessie. However, you will often find that grocery stores put the egg cartons in the same refrigerated section as the milk cartons, so we've put them here as well. Everything you need to know in order to make an educated egg purchase can be found in the flurry of information—and misinformation—on the front of the egg cartons themselves. Why does one egg say natural, while another claims organic? What is the difference between cage-free, pastured, and free-range chickens? The manufacturers have created so many terms, but what do they actually mean, and which eggs should you choose?

Remember, we want to avoid foods that have been raised with unnatural feed and environments (EMD). So, in order to figure out what we should be looking for in the healthiest eggs, we need to understand what our feathered friends prefer and what is natural for chickens. First, chickens like to roam and spread their wings, not live in cages with prohibitive space to move. Additionally, it is important to recognize that chickens are omnivores. They just love greens and bugs and enjoy a good day of hunting and pecking in the dirt to forage for their food.

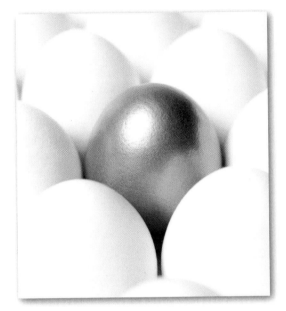

So where do you find chickens that lay the golden eggs? Here we steer you out of the supermarket and to your local farm or farmers market. The gold standard for eggs is to have been raised on fresh pastures and allowed both their natural feed and environment. According to *Mother Earth News* magazine, eggs from pastured flocks contain two times more omega-3 fatty acids, four to six times more vitamin D, two-thirds more vitamin A, three times more vitamin E, and seven times more beta-carotene than conventional factory farmed eggs. Another study in the *British Journal of Nutrition* found that pastured hen eggs had 170 percent more energy-boosting B12 and 150 percent more folate than their confined commercial counterparts.

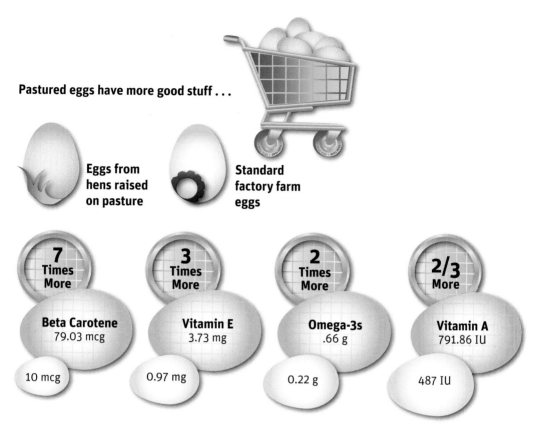

Pastured eggs have more good stuff . . .

Eggs from hens raised on pasture

Standard factory farm eggs

7 Times More

Beta Carotene
79.03 mcg

10 mcg

3 Times More

Vitamin E
3.73 mg

0.97 mg

2 Times More

Omega-3s
.66 g

0.22 g

2/3 More

Vitamin A
791.86 IU

487 IU

If you are sticking to supermarket shopping, here are some common carton callouts that can help to determine egg-xactly which eggs to buy!

USDA Certified Organic

These happy hens must be fed organic, non-GMO feed, free of both antibiotics and pesticides. Additionally, the chickens must be kept uncaged in barns or warehouses, and it is required that they have outdoor access (although no time minimum is mandated). Unlike organic cows, which must have some access to grass, there are no guidelines mandating that organic chickens be let out on grass at all. While the added vitamin D they absorb from sunshine is beneficial, it would be preferred if their environment was more natural than an enclosed porch or concrete slab.

CERTIFIED

Pasture-raised

While this term is unregulated, it implies that the chickens were raised receiving at least some time—the more the better—roaming free in pastures. Allowing our feathered friends their natural environment supplies the birds with their natural diet of both vegetation and critters, which then supplies you with a better, more micronutrient-rich egg.

DAIRY

Cage-free

The USDA says this label means that chickens are kept out of cages and have continuous access to food and water but generally have no access to the outdoors. While they can spread their wings, both their environment and their feed have been altered. These closeted clucks can't peck around in the dirt for bugs—not exactly the perfect conditions for our poultry.

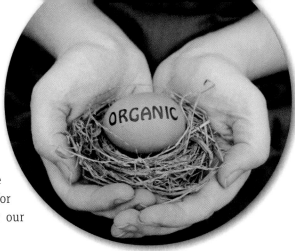

Free-range

While free-range means something on some poultry products, there are no guidelines or standards that must be met on egg cartons. Free-range hens are much like the cage-free birds, imprisoned in warehouses and barns. However, they must have exhibited some good behavior because these inmates get some yard time—although much like real humans doing jail time, yard time may often be nothing more than a concrete lot to enjoy for a few minutes a day. These un-cheery chickens are still left only fantasizing about the freedom to roam free, peck, and eat.

100 Percent Vegetarian-fed

What? Chickens aren't vegetarians —they like bugs, so this claim screams foul for the poor fowl! Chickens that eat only diets of vegetarian feed don't eat their natural diet and produce eggs that are depleted of their essential micronutrients. However, when the carton says 100 percent vegetarian feed, you are guaranteed that your chickens did not eat animal by-products in their feed, and this is, of course, a good thing. We crack up when labels claim their chickens are pastured and vegetarian. Can you imagine why? What did the farmer do, tie shut the chicken's beaks to make sure the hens didn't peck in the dirt and eat bugs when they were out in the pasture? As you can see, the manufacturers who put these two claims together haven't a clue about their clucks.

United Egg Producers Certified

Don't be fooled by this certification. The overwhelming majority of the US egg industry complies with this inhumane, voluntary program, where the average hen is crammed into a cage only as large as a sheet of paper.

No Hormones

This is meaningless as the USDA never approved any hormone products for egg production.

Natural or Naturally Raised

Empty statement meant to induce images of wide-open pastures.

Omega-3

How do chickens end up with greater amounts of the omega-3 fatty acids believed to improve heart health and memory? Farmers either pasture their birds or add sources of omega-3s, such as flaxseed or algae, to their diets. Either way, these extra omegas are egg-xtra beneficial.

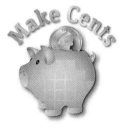

Pasture-raised, organic eggs are the best, but purchasing them at the grocery store can cost you. So venture out to the local farm or farmers market where you can pick them up dirt cheap. Not all small farms can afford the organic certification, but don't let that deter you. Visit the farm whenever possible, ask questions, and determine for yourself if they are following all the organic guidelines. If they are, pick up a dozen. Make cents?

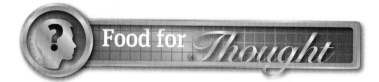

Look no further. The incredible, edible egg may just be the most perfect diet food available. Two St. Louis University studies determined that eating an egg in the morning while dieting improved weight loss by 65 percent, while reducing appetite throughout the day. This may be due to all the fantastic essential micronutrients hidden just beneath the egg's fragile shell. Eggs supply iodine for good thyroid function. (Low iodine levels can cause weight gain and lethargy.) The high levels of vitamin D in eggs fight cancer and help to build strong bones. It bears repeating: vitamin D-deficient women have been shown to be on average 16.3 pounds heavier than sufficient women. Eggs also contain choline, which is a natural fat emulsifier. And don't forget about the omega-3.

Gettysburg College studies determined that adding omega-3 to one's diet significantly lowers cortisol levels. By reducing this cortisol, which increases fat deposits in the belly and suppresses immune function, the subjects were able to shed three-and-a-half times more body fat, while increasing lean muscle mass. If you are on a diet, it's time to get cracking!

If your low-fat diet tells you to eat only the white, you may want to reconsider. That yellow yolk contains 100 percent of the fat-soluble vitamins A, D, E, and K, as well as all of the carotenoids lutein and zeaxanthin found in the egg. It also contains more than 90 percent of the calcium, iron, phosphorus, zinc, thiamin, folate, vitamin B6, and vitamin B12. Indeed, egg yolks are among the most micronutrient-dense foods on the planet, while eggs whites are merely a moderately good source of protein. Forget the "Egg Beaters"—nothing beats real, pasture-raised eggs!

DAIRY

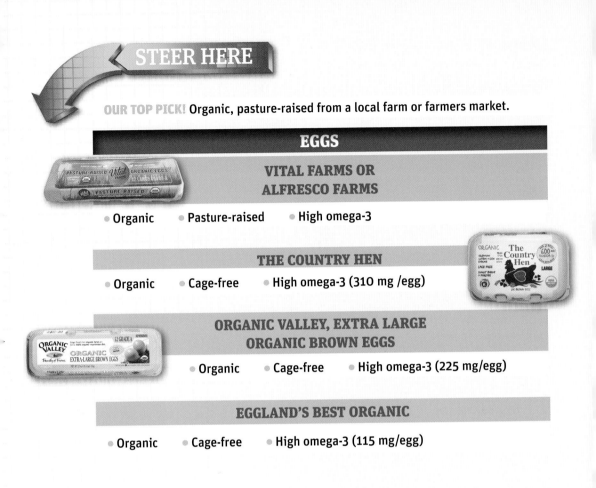

OUR TOP PICK! Organic, pasture-raised from a local farm or farmers market.

EGGS

VITAL FARMS OR ALFRESCO FARMS

- Organic
- Pasture-raised
- High omega-3

THE COUNTRY HEN

- Organic
- Cage-free
- High omega-3 (310 mg /egg)

ORGANIC VALLEY, EXTRA LARGE ORGANIC BROWN EGGS

- Organic
- Cage-free
- High omega-3 (225 mg/egg)

EGGLAND'S BEST ORGANIC

- Organic
- Cage-free
- High omega-3 (115 mg/egg)

GREAT VALUE LIQUID EGGS

This troublesome time saver actually adds sugar, in the form of GMO maltodextrin, into your omelet. Use real eggs, which are still intact.

ALL POWDERED EGGS

Powdered eggs should always be avoided because they are a source of unwanted oxidized cholesterol. Unlike cholesterol, which itself is not dangerous, cholesterol that has been oxidized is far more prone to form plaque in the walls of arteries. *CAUTION:* When staying at hotels or eating at restaurants, choose fried eggs over scrambled. Restaurants and budget buffets often use these cheap powdered eggs when they aren't presented whole such as with scrambled eggs or in recipes calling for eggs.

□ Choose organic eggs or eggs purchased from a farm that follows the organic guidelines.

□ Choose pastured eggs.

□ Choose free-range or cage-free eggs when pastured aren't possible.

□ Choose eggs with high omega-3 content.

□ Avoid meaningless claims like natural, no hormones, and United Egg Producers Certified.

□ Avoid all eggs that are not in shells, including all liquid or powdered eggs.

*My go-to Rich Food choices for eggs:*_____

_____

_____

_____

_____

_____

_____

_____

_____

_____

_____

_____

_____

Aisle

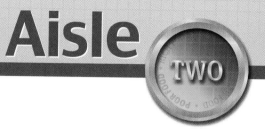

TWO

Meat

A s we continue around the perimeter of the supermarket in search of Rich Foods, our next stop is the meat department. Much like the deceptive labeling on boxed, bagged, and bottled products in other aisles, the meat department is a minefield of confusing, purposely ambiguous labels (remember the misleading misfits from Chapter 3) and hidden ingredients.

Fresh from the Butcher

WE LONG FOR THE DAYS of the mom-and-pop butcher shops with sawdust on the floor and chops hanging in the backdrop. While they might not be popular these days, the butchers in your grocer's meat department are highly knowledgeable and ready to help you on your quest toward Rich Food meat choices. If you don't already know your butchers by name, we suggest you get to know them. They can lead you to the best cuts of meat. However, they may not be able to help you choose the healthiest, most micronutrient-rich source of meat—that's what we are here for.

Whether you are looking for a heavily marbled rib-eye or a fat-trimmed chicken breast, the manner in which an animal is raised makes a big difference in its overall ability to deliver a delicious, healthy meal. The great news for all you animal lovers out there is that the happier and more humanely treated animals are, the healthier and more micronutrient-rich they are. So take a stand and choose meat from animals that were treated humanely. Gratefully, there are some terrific organizations acting as watchdogs, making sure animals are treated well.

Look for these logos to identify the good guys looking out for our health as well as the health of the livestock.

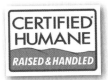 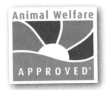 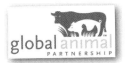

CERTIFIED HUMANE:	AMERICAN HUMANE CERTIFIED:	ANIMAL WELFARE APPROVED:	GLOBAL ANIMAL PARTNERSHIP:
A certification and label program developed by Humane Farm Animal Care and endorsed by the ASPCA and other humane organizations.	A program of the American Humane Association.	Run by the Animal Welfare Institute, the newest and currently the strictest certification and labeling program.	A 5-step program used by Whole Foods Market that aims to improve the welfare of agricultural animals.

The Grass Grazers

ALTHOUGH COWS, BISON, SHEEP, DEER, AND GOAT all appear to be quite different from one another, they have one important thing in common—they're all ruminants, which means that they eat plant-based diets and digest them through the process of "rumination"— chewing, regurgitation, and rechewing cud to stimulate digestion. Their natural, grass-fed diets have traditionally supplied them with all the nutrients they need to produce micronutrient-rich steaks and chops. Unfortunately, today's conventional farms (aka CAFOs—Concentrated Animal

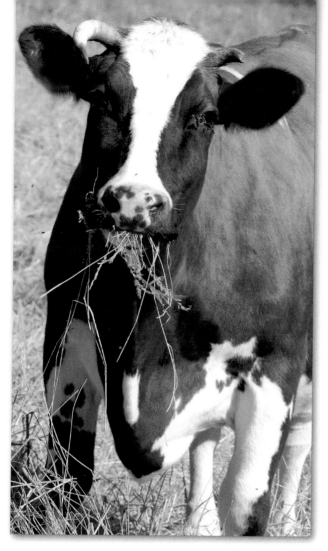

Feeding Operations) want to hurry the process along, so rather than allow these animals the time to graze on grasses as they freely roam the pastures, animals are locked in confined spaces and fed diets full of GMO grain. While the feed, filled with antibiotics and growth hormones, increases their size rapidly, it also causes the animals to endure many health problems. Unfortunately, these unhealthy CAFO animals comprise the vast majority of meat available in the grocery story today. If it's not labeled otherwise, you can bet that your meat comes from undesirable CAFO production.

So, if you are like us and want to avoid these factory-farmed meats, what should you look for? How do you identify the most robust ruminants? The following are a few terms to help you analyze the Angus.

Grass-Fed

To be labeled grass-fed, the USDA requires that the animals were raised on a lifetime diet of 100 percent grass and forage (with the exception of milk consumed prior to weaning). Unlike the term *organic*, however, it does not exclude the use of antibiotics, hormones, or pesticides or disallow the use of GMO grasses—which can include corn, soybean, rice, wheat, and oats in their pre-grain, vegetative state. Still, these grass-feeders supply us with more micronutrient-rich meats, containing higher levels of healthy fats like CLA and omega-3 and lower amounts of omega-6 and saturated fat than grain-fed cows.

Additionally, grass-fed lamb is 14 percent lower in fat, is 8 percent higher in protein, and has twice as much lutein (which reduces the risk of macular degeneration, a leading cause of blindness) as their grain-fed counterparts. Grass-fed bison has more than four times the amount of vitamin E as grain-fed counterparts.

MEAT

Don't be fooled by companies that state their cows are *pastured*. These cows may have been *in* a pasture at some point, but more than likely, they were also fed grains if the words *grass-fed* do not appear prominently on the label. If you see the following grass-fed symbols on the label, you can be sure that their living conditions have been examined and certified as healthy.

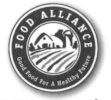

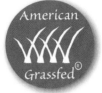

USDA PROCESS VERIFIED SHIELD: verifies animals were raised on a lifetime diet of 100 percent grass and forage.

FOOD ALLIANCE: verifies animals were raised on a lifetime diet of 100 percent grass and forage. Additionally, meats carrying this symbol are certified for not using antibiotics or hormones.

AMERICAN GRASSFED ASSOCIATION: verifies animals were raised on a lifetime diet of 100 percent grass and forage without confinement, antibiotics, or hormones.

Grass-finished

The manner cattle are fed in the last few weeks or months before processing determines how an animal is "finished." Grass-fed meat should be finished on grass; however, some farms grain finish to improve taste and texture as well as hasten the maturation and harvesting process. During the time of grass finishing, the levels of important nutrients like cancer-fighting, fat-metabolizing CLA and inflammation-reducing omega-3 increase dramatically in the beef. That is why it's so important to make sure that the beef you eat is not only grass-fed, but grass-finished. You can be guaranteed the cattle was grass-finished by choosing beef verified by the grass-fed organizations above. The term *100 percent grass-fed* is often used to distinguish between a naturally raised animal and one that endured a grain-fed approach to the finish line.

Organic

Purchasing organic beef guarantees that your meat is free of antibiotics, hormones, and GMOs. These animals must also have time to pasture, but it is minimal (120 days) and the vast majority of what they eat (up to 70 percent) is permitted to come from non-GMO grains that are difficult for the animals to process. While you are minimizing your toxic load, you are not guaranteed the greater micronutrient levels of grazing ruminants. Choose a labeled grass-fed organic meat to be sure you are buying only the best.

A Medley of Meats

DO YOU GET SICK OF SERVING UP the same dinners night after night? Round up some new ruminant choices for your clan!

Lamb

While beef is America's darling, leg of lamb is Australia's national dish. To choose the freshest cut of lamb from the butcher, look for the pinkest flesh. To avoid a gamier taste, choose leaner cuts, as much of that flavor is held in the fat.

Goat

You may be shocked to learn that goat is the world's most-consumed meat, making up almost 70 percent of the red meat eaten globally. Not true grazers, goats are considered "browsers" and will try to eat almost anything. While they may sample many things, goats are quite particular in what they actually consume, preferring the flavors of woody shrubs and trees. Try goat for a lean, savory meat that works well with spicy and sour flavors.

Bison

These magnificent animals are the largest native land mammals in North America. Bison meat, also known as buffalo, has 33 percent more protein, 14 percent more iron, and 8 percent more B12 than beef. This leaner, lower calorie option offers a taste that is similar to that of a fine cut of beef, with a bit sweeter and more robust flavor.

Don't see these cuts at your grocery store? Talk to your butcher about placing a special order.

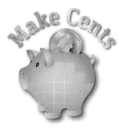

From its strips to its tips, grass-fed organic beef can cost you. If you want to save money and you love steaks, burgers, and ribs, consider putting an energy-efficient freezer in your garage or basement. While it may cost you up to fifty dollars a year to keep it cold, you'll save money by buying your meat in bulk.

Did you know that you can buy a whole cow, or as little as an eighth of a cow, directly from a farm? When you do, you pay one single price per pound. You can get a great assortment of cuts to enjoy for close to the cost of the grass-fed ground beef (the cheapest cut) in the grocery store. To find a farm in your area, visit our Rich Food Resource Center online. Is the farm too far from the house? Don't have the time? Talk to neighbors or coworkers and share the burden.

Remember, just because a farmer, whether local or a nationwide wholesaler, has not applied for their organic certification, does not mean that he or she isn't following all the guidelines. Ask questions. Be an educated shopper. Many times, the certification is too expensive for the farms, but they are doing a great job raising healthy animals. You can be assured that we've put our Rich Food choices to the test!

MEAT

Chicken and Turkey

WHEN CHOOSING the best chickens for soups, parmesans, or cacciatore, we can use much of the same information that we have already learned when choosing eggs in the dairy aisle. As we stated earlier, chickens are omnivores, so the most nutritious poultry picks are those that are allowed to spend time in pastures eating both grass and insects. This may seem quite simple, but the manufacturers will throw you some curveballs by labeling chickens with a slew of slippery terms—those misleading misfits . . . again.

Natural

This term only guarantees that there are no artificial colors, flavors, or preservatives and that the bird has been "minimally processed." This does not mean that the poultry isn't pumped up with a salt solution, often labeled as added solution or "enhanced water." Federal law allows water absorption in poultry of up to 12 percent. You pay the same amount for that water as you do for the bird. That is some expensive aqua!

Free-range

While this term meant absolutely nothing on the egg carton, it means only slightly more for the poultry. According to the USDA, a mere five minutes of open air access per day is required for a bird to receive free-range status. Remember, *open air* can still mean *enclosed in a concrete pen with nowhere to hunt and peck.*

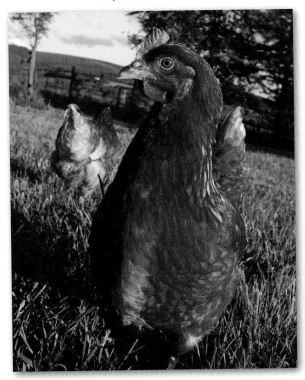

Hormone Free/No Added Hormones

US law prohibits the use of growth hormones in poultry. So, when you see this on the label, you should know that the company is simply boasting about the fact that they are not breaking the law by meeting government standards.

Antibiotic Free/No Antibiotics

US law does allow antibiotics, so when you see this on a label, it means the bird you're buying didn't receive antibiotics at any time. Chickens who fall ill and are administered antibiotics are not eligible for this status.

Raised without the Routine Use of Antibiotics

This means that antibiotics may have been administered for illness but not as a preventative measure.

Pastured or Pasture Raised

Now we are getting somewhere. Like pastured eggs, pastured poultry wins the prize! These birds boast higher micronutrient density due to their healthier diets; however, it is still important to make sure that your pastured birds are organic. This is because, unlike cows, who thrive on grass alone, chickens must still get some of their food from feed mixes—often as high as 50 percent— which can include corn, soybeans, alfalfa, clover, and oats. Only by choosing organic chickens can you be sure that the feed is free of GMOs.

Air Chilled

This is a relatively new term that refers not to how a bird is bred, but rather to how it is processed. Most chickens, prior to packaging, are taken to chillers or community-style chlorine baths, into which each day's birds go in and out. With air chilling, the birds are not mixed together in these community baths. This results in bacteria counts that are 80 percent lower than those of water-chilled chickens. Additionally, the birds don't absorb extra water before packaging, which means you are not charged for this extra weight in the grocery store. Finally, these birds just taste better. Unlike water-chilled birds that lose their natural flavorful juices as the water escapes during cooking, air-chilled birds lock in more chickeny goodness.

Organic

According to USDA standards, organic poultry must be fed 100 percent organic, non-GMO feed that contains no animal by-products. It also must be free of pesticide, chemical fertilizers, hormones, and antibiotics. They must receive outdoor access but no duration or location requirements are indicated. Additionally, organic poultry cannot suffer micronutrient loss due to irradiation.

MEAT

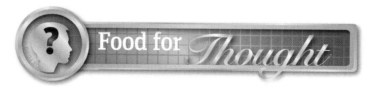

According to the FDA, poultry farmers are permitted to feed arsenic, a recognized carcinogen to birds, for "growth promotion, feed efficiency, and improved pigmentation." The arsenic affects the blood vessels in chickens and turkeys, causing them to appear pinker and therefore fresher. When the Institute for Agriculture and Trade Policy, a Minnesota-based advocacy group, tested conventional poultry, it found the poison in 55 percent of chicken parts (breast, thighs, and livers) tested, with the highest amount—21.2 parts per *million*—occurring in generic brands. If you want to know how safe that is, you should know that the EPA considers 10 parts per *billion* in drinking water to be high enough to pose a cancer risk. The chickens tested had up to two thousand times more of these cancer-causing arsenic levels! The European Union has outlawed the use of arsenic since 1999, and you should ban it from your body by choosing organic birds.

In 2012, scientists from Johns Hopkins University tested poultry from six states and China to determine the chemical exposures. They found arsenic in 100 percent of the samples collected. Unfortunately, arsenic was not the only unwanted chemical lurking in the non-organic poultry. The majority of samples also contained acetaminophen, the active ingredient in Tylenol, and one-third of the samples contained the antihistamine used in Benadryl. The samples from China also showed traces of Prozac, most likely administered to the chickens to reduce the stress of their poor living conditions. But that is not the worst of it! The most troubling substance identified was a broad-spectrum class of antibiotics called fluoroquinolones, which the FDA banned for poultry production back in 2005. While some antibiotics are allowed in non-organic poultry to reduce infections and rapidly increase a bird's size, this particular class of drugs breeds so-called superbugs, which cause antibiotic-resistant infections in humans. This means that many years after the ban went into effect, this illegal antibiotic is still being detected in non-organic poultry. So that big bird is a really big problem!

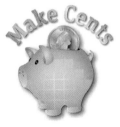

To save money when purchasing organic, pastured birds, buy the birds whole. Chicken breasts, thighs, and legs cost far more when pre-packaged into pieces. For the price of a couple of breasts, you can get a whole bird.

If organic pastured birds are still price prohibitive, here are some tips for purchasing conventional clucks.

- **BUY THE BREAST.** Leaner cuts will contain fewer toxins, as toxins are more concentrated in the animal's fat.
- **CHOOSE BIRDS LABELED TO HAVE RECEIVED 100 PERCENT VEGE-TARIAN FEED.** While we recognize that these birds are omnivores, this phrase protects the caged clucks from being fed animal by-products.

Pork—the Other White Meat

PIGS, LIKE CHICKENS, ARE OMNIVORES, which means their natural diet would include grass, leafy greens, nuts, fruits, and roots, as well as animals, most often insects. However, when confined in factory farms, in cages no larger than their plump exteriors, they are commonly fed genetically modified corn and soybean meal, growth hormones, and antibiotics. Pastured pigs that are also fed organic diets are our pick because these humanely raised animals produce meat with lower levels of saturated fat and higher levels of vitamin E, selenium, and heart-healthy omega-3. Watch out if buying conventional pork products. Ninety percent of supermarket pork is up to 40 percent water.

The World's Most Loved Pork Product—Bacon

The cut of meat used to prepare bacon varies by region. In the United States, it is almost always prepared from pork belly, which gives it its fatty, streaked appearance. The traditional bacon of the UK and Canada is back bacon, a far leaner cut taken from the back loin. While the cut may alter the strip's fat content, we want to draw your attention to the curing process. Traditionally, only hams were cured with added white or brown sugar, honey, or molasses. It is unfortunate that almost all store-bought brands of bacon today add sugar to the cure. While this is common, it is unnecessary. Purchasing pork belly or bacon from a local farmer and salt curing it yourself may be your best bet to ensure sugar has not been added.

Deli Meat Disasters

DO YOU BUY PREPACKAGED sliced meats or hand-sliced meats from your supermarket's deli department? Regardless of where your sandwich meat is purchased, the same factors need to be considered. First, terms like *pastured, grass-fed,* and *organic* are as important to look for as they are in the meats discussed above. However, many of these sliced sandwich meats come with some new added Poor Food ingredients that you may not be looking for, including sugar, corn syrup, synthetic nitrates, and non-organic (irradiated) spices (we will discuss spices further in Aisle 7: Baking).

While you can easily see these unwanted add-ins on the ingredient list of the prepackaged deli meats, you will have to ask the counter clerk in the deli department to look for an unopened, still labeled package to tell you what lurks in the ingredient list.

Also, unless you want to be paying the same price per pound for water as you are for meat, avoid meats that have water included in the ingredient list. While not all sliced sandwich meats fall into our Poor Food pit, most do. Ideally, you want to see just the meat on the ingredient list,

MEAT

and perhaps some organic spices. If you really love deli meat, it may be better to invest in a small meat slicer and slice up your grass-fed or pastured organic meats yourself.

Our Ancestor's Favorite Meat Was Offal!

HAVE YOU EVER WONDERED what cut of meat our ancestors prized above all others? What were the tribal leaders and revered warriors given to eat after a successful hunt? Well, anthropologists indicate that it wasn't a fat-free chicken breast. In many cultures, it was offal (pronounced "awful")—the internal organs of the animal. Our ancestors coveted bits of liver, heart, kidneys, brains, and intestines, slathered in a sauce of warm blood. After the truly offal stuff (sorry, couldn't resist!), ribs and backbone were the next choices, followed last but not least by the muscle meats—the stuff we pay the most for today!

What they knew—and what we seem to have forgotten—is that these organ meats are by far the most micronutrient-dense parts of the animal. Liver, for instance, is an excellent source of the fat-soluble vitamins A and K2, as well as folate, selenium, vitamin B12, and copper; it also has high levels of CoQ10, potassium, vitamin D, and heme iron. Heart is rich in thiamin, folate, selenium, phosphorus, zinc, and CoQ10. You get the point. While we are not suggesting you trade your filet mignon in for tripe, adding some organic, grass-fed organ meats into your diet is a marvelous way to boost your micronutrient level.

Not sure how to incorporate offal into your current diet? If you are like most people, your first few attempts with offal may scare you a bit—it did us! But we guarantee that the benefits are huge,

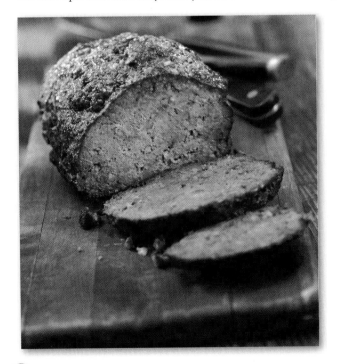

and by following our directions, you won't even know it is in the recipe. Liver may be the easiest to start with, but don't just fry up a plate of liver and onions if you are a newbie—and don't even tell your family you are sneaking it in if you are the chef! Our favorite way to incorporate liver into our diet is to first get the freshest liver you can find (as instructed above) and then blend it in a blender—literally liquefying the liver. From here, the sky is the limit; you can use it in any recipe where you use ground beef. You can try meatballs, meatloaf, chili, or our favorite: a spicy

Mexican beef dip! Add in 1 part liver to 3 parts grass-fed beef. Adjust the ratio to fit your recipe's needs. You will also need to "beef up" the spice content. Remember to use organic spices to avoid the free radicals caused by irradiation (more in Aisle 7: Baking). Live it up! Liven your dinner with liver. We bet your family won't even know you've done it—our guests never do!

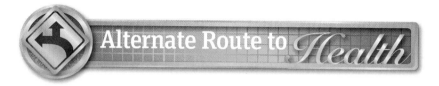

Park your shopping cart and find your way to the farm. As we stated earlier, shopping for your meats directly from local farmers can mean big savings to you. But the real reason for purchasing your proteins in person is your health. You can visit the farms and see for yourself how the animals are raised. Are the pigs' snouts covered in mud from spending happy days routing for roots? Do the chickens have ample space to nest and peck? Pick up the feedbags and see for yourself if they are GMO free. This way, you can be assured that the animals are being raised within their natural environments, eating their natural feeds, which in turns supplies you with the safest, most micronutrient-rich meat (not) on the market.

Make No Bones About It—Bone Broth Is the Original *Souper*food

WONDERING WHAT TO DO WITH THE BONES from the high-quality protein you just enjoyed for dinner? Don't toss them in the trash. There is life in those old bones yet. The broth you make from bones too often discarded can create a health tonic with numerous benefits. Not only is soup comforting to the soul, it is incredibly nourishing to the body. First, bone broth contains easily absorbable forms of minerals such as calcium, silicon, sulphur, magnesium, and phosphorous. The gelatin in bone broth (unlike the hydrolyzed form that may contain MSG and is often added to packaged foods) assists digestion by attracting digestive juices and has also been shown to help heal prior damage to the gut lining, offering relief for those with Irritable Bowel Syndrome (IBS), Crohn's disease, and other digestive disorders. A bowl of broth also contains chondroitin sulfate, now famous as a supplement for osteoarthritic joint pain. The amino acid proline in bone broth has been shown to play an important role in combatting arteriosclerosis, or hardening of the arteries, by allowing for the release of fat buildup into the bloodstream, decreasing blockages and thus reducing risk of heart disease. This same elixir can have fantastic effects on your outside as well, because the collagen in bone broth helps smooth your skin and prevents wrinkles and cellulite. Have we sold you on this *souper*food yet?

MEAT

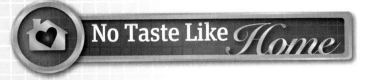

Don't settle for store-bought broth. Most boxes and canned varieties add in unwanted Poor Food ingredients, most often sweeteners, gluten, and preservatives. Use this recipe to make a far more nutritious option at home. It freezes perfectly, so you can just pop some out of the freezer whenever you run out. Use it as a base for soups, to sauté, or drink it alone for all of its incredible health benefits.

So Simple Souperfood

INGREDIENTS:

- Bones (You can use raw or cooked chicken carcasses, marrow bones from the butcher, ribs, etc. Try to use the bones from quality-grass fed/pasture raised proteins.)
- 2–3 Tbsp. organic apple cider vinegar
- Garlic, chopped at least 15 minutes before heating
- Unrefined sea salt (see our guide in Aisle 7: Baking)
- Filtered water

DIRECTIONS:

1 Place all ingredients in a slow cooker. Make sure the water is high enough to cover the bones. Do not forget to add the vinegar. This is the ingredient that pulls the minerals from the bones.

2 Bring to a boil, and then reduce to low heat.

3 Remember, patience is a virtue. The longer you let your broth brew, the better it will be. Leave chicken broth in a slow cooker for 24 hours and beef broth up to 48 hours.

 4 Turn heat off and allow it to cool.

 5 Strain the cooled broth using a cheesecloth or fine mesh metal strainer. Keep only the liquid.

 6 Refrigerate. Once cooled, it may form a thick waxy layer of fat (tallow) on the surface. Skim it off, and either toss it or save it for cooking.

You can store your soup safely in the refrigerator for up to four days. Better yet, place some in the freezer to keep for later use. You can enjoy a simple mug of bone broth to warm you up on a cool day, or use it as your starter for soups. Add vegetables, meat, and grain-free pastas for a heartier soup. You can even enjoy it for breakfast like they do in many Asian countries. Add bits of meat and veggies, a few spices, and our zughetti (see page 189), and you have yourself a delicious and nutritious bowl of Vietnamese pho—one of our favorite ways to start the day.

STEER HERE

OUR TOP PICK! Organic, 100 percent pasture-raised or grass-fed meats from a local farm or reputable butcher.

GRASS-FED BEEF

WHITE OAK GRASS-FED BEEF

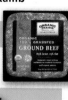

- Grass-fed and grass-finished • No GMO feed
- No synthetic hormones • No antibiotics
- Humane Farm Animal Care endorsement
- Animal Welfare Approved • American Grassfed Association endorsement
- Global Animal Partnership endorsement • Also supplies exceptional lamb

ORGANIC PRAIRIE PREMIUM GRASS FED BEEF

- Grass-fed and grass-finished • Organic

JONES CREEK BEEF

- Grass-fed and grass-finished beef
- No synthetic hormones • No antibiotics

THOUSAND HILLS CATTLE COMPANY

- Grass-fed and grass-finished • No GMO feed • No synthetic hormones
- No antibiotics

HEARST RANCH BEEF

- Grass-fed and grass-finished • No GMO feed • No synthetic hormones
- No antibiotics • Food Alliance Certified
- Also serving incredible lamb and pork products

SOMMERS ORGANIC GRASS-FED BEEF

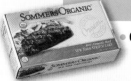

- Grass-fed (although it doesn't say so on the package) • Organic

IN THE FREEZER

APPLEGATE ORGANICS ORGANIC BEEF BURGERS

- Grass-fed and grass-finished • Organic

MEAT

LAMB

ATKINS RANCH

- Grass-fed and grass-finished
- Organic

HEARST RANCH LAMB

- Grass-fed and grass-finished
- No GMO feed
- No synthetic hormones
- No antibiotics
- Food Alliance Certified

POULTRY

PETALUMA POULTRY "ROSIE" ORGANIC FREE RANGE CHICKENS

- Organic
- Free-range

MARY'S FREE RANGE, AIR CHILLED, ORGANIC CHICKEN AND FREE RANGE ORGANIC TURKEYS

- Organic
- Free range
- Air chilled
- Global Animal Partnership

While we recommend this option, we do not recommend their pasture-raised chicken and turkey because their birds are not certified organic, which indicates to us that they may be using GMO feed, pesticides, antibiotics, or chemical fertilizers.

ORGANIC BELL & EVANS AIR CHILLED POULTRY

- Organic
- Free range
- Air chilled

They even have organic chicken wings that are perfect for your next party!

PORK

BECKER LANE ORGANIC FARMS

- Organic
- Pasture raised
- Animal Welfare approved

Look for their acorn-finished pork products around the holidays.

THOMPSON FARMS

- Pasture raised
- No GMO feed
- No synthetic hormones
- No antibiotics
- Global Animal Partnership

DELI

WEGMANS ORGANIC FOOD YOU FEEL GOOD ABOUT GRASS-FED ROAST BEEF

- Organic
- Grass-fed

GRATEFUL HARVEST ORGANIC DELI MEATS

- Organic
- Grass-fed roast beef
- Their turkey, chicken, and ham are all sugar free.

APPLEGATE FARMS DELI COUNTER NO SALT OR WATER ADDED TURKEY

- No synthetic hormones
- No antibiotics

ONLINE OPTIONS
(look for links in the Rich Food Resource Center online)

U.S. WELLNESS MEATS

They sell it all. And the best part is that it all ships at once, stocking your freezer with an assortment of the best quality meat. Wow! They sell some of the only sugar-free, GMO-free, pasture-raised bacon we have ever found.

GREENSBURY MARKET

USDA certified organic 100 percent grass-fed and grass-finished beef, and organic pastured chicken and pork. Animal Welfare approved.

TROPICAL TRADITIONS

Pastured organic chickens and turkeys, raised with a coconut-based, soy-free, non-GMO feed called coco feed. They also carry 100 percent grass-fed and grass-finished bison, beef, and lamb.

BROKEN ARROW RANCH

It is time to break out of the ordinary. This ranch is an artisanal purveyor of high-quality, free-range venison, antelope, and boar meat from truly wild animals. Go wild at the dinner table!

Note: You may notice that we didn't label our organic choices as free of GMO feed, synthetic hormones, and antibiotics. Remember, these facts are true of all organic products. Keep this in mind as we move through the aisles.

MEAT

BEEF

CONVENTIONAL GROUND BEEF

Besides the obvious GMO feed, antibiotics, and hormones these cattle endure, 50 percent of conventional grocery store brands contain undesirable pink slime (a mechanically separated melting pot of mixed meat pieces) that's received some unwanted national media attention recently.

BALL PARK BRAND FROZEN FLAME GRILLED BEEF PATTIES

First, we begin with a poor quality, GMO-fed ground beef, likely loaded with hormones, pesticides, and antibiotics. While Ball Park promised to leave out the pink slime, they did load up their patties with water (expensive weight increaser), dextrose and maltodextrin (GMO corn sweeteners), partially hydroge-nated soybean oil (GMO trans fat), and yeast extract (MSG). With more than three strikes, they are out of the cart.

POULTRY

CONVENTIONAL CHICKEN

Avoid the dark meats for their higher levels of numerous toxins.

HILLSHIRE FARM'S GRILLED CHICKEN BREAST

This seemingly simple chicken breast contains more than twenty ingredients, including partially hydrogenated GMO oils (trans fats), hydrolyzed corn protein (MSG), and dextrose (GMO sugar).

PORK

FARMLAND BACON, HONEY & MAPLE FLAVORED NATURALLY HICKORY SMOKED

Poor-quality pork swimming in a sea of honey, maple syrup, sugar, nitrites, and caramel color.

HORMEL EXTRA LEAN PORK TENDERLOIN ORIGINAL FLAVOR

Up to 30 percent of what you are purchasing with this pork is a water solution that contains partially hydrogenated soybean oil (GMO trans fat), autolyzed yeast (MSG), and cornstarch (GMO).

DELI

OSCAR MAYER HAM AND CHEDDAR LUNCHABLES

There are sixty-one ingredients in this offensive offering. Poor quality meat (ham chopped and formed with artificial flavors and added water) packaged with crackers (labeled *made with* whole grain) and a "vanilla cream cookie" containing neither vanilla nor cream.

ARMOUR DELI BOLOGNA

Imagine the scraps a butcher might give to his dog after a long day of packaging chickens, turkeys, beef, and pork. Now, toss it all together in a blender, mix in some MSG, nitrites, and assorted GMO corn sweeteners, and throw it in a mold to give a new, perfectly round silhouette. Stick the Armour label on it, and enjoy your Poor Food, mechanically separated meat masterpiece.

HORMEL NATURAL CHOICE 100% NATURAL CANADIAN BACON

One of the worst deli meats we found. What looks like sliced Canadian bacon contains more than thirty ingredients, including sugar, molasses, corn syrup, brown sugar, honey, pineapple juice concentrate, hydrolyzed soy protein, hydrolyzed corn gluten, caramel color, wheat starch, soy flour, and soybean oil.

CAUTION FOR COOKS

SOME STUDIES SHOW that cooking meats at high temperatures can cause heterocyclic amines (HCAs) and polycyclic aromatic hydrocarbons (PAHs) to form. Both of these formations have been linked to colorectal cancer, prostate cancer, and breast cancer. They get into your food when dripping meat juices cause the grilling surface or coals to flare up; while the flames are adding flavor, they are also engulfing the meat or fish in toxic vapors.

Here are some tips to guarantee you a safer grill:

1 Turn down the heat and raise the rack. Temperatures over 300 degrees Fahrenheit trigger HCA formation.

2 Turn with tongs. Using a fork can puncture the meat, which causes drippings to flare up the flame.

3 Flip meat frequently. Turning every few minutes has been shown to greatly reduce HCAs.

4 Avoid overcooking. Chargrilled pieces contain the most toxins. Cut off any charred sections.

5 Marinate your meat. Recently, scientists at the Food Safety Consortium project at Kansas State University discovered that when marinades were made with herbs such as basil, mint, rosemary, thyme, oregano, and sage, HCA formation was reduced by up to 99 percent.

MEAT

- ☐ Choose organic meats.
- ☐ Choose grass-fed and grass-finished ruminants and pastured poultry and pigs.
- ☐ Choose air-chilled chicken.
- ☐ Choose whole chickens to save money.
- ☐ Choose white meat that is fed a 100 percent vegetarian feed when purchasing conventional (non-organic) chicken.
- ☐ Choose to purchase grass-fed and grass-finished meats from local farmers in bulk to save money (e.g., 1/8 steer or 1/4 pig).
- ☐ Choose organic deli meats with the fewest ingredients.
- ☐ Avoid products that add in extra water.
- ☐ Avoid animals raised inhumanely in factory farms/feedlots.
- ☐ Avoid MSG under all its aliases.
- ☐ Avoid sweeteners and all GMO additives (corn and soy).
- ☐ Avoid charring your meat when cooking.
- ☐ Avoid all packaged meat flavored with solutions, "enhanced waters," or in prepackage marinades to avoid paying for expensive water with added sodium and potential MSG.

My go-to Rich Food choices for meats : _____

_____

_____

_____

_____

_____

_____

_____

Hot Dog! Brats and Sausage, Too.

It is no secret that when it comes to nutritional value, this summer favorite has got a bad *wrap*—and we aren't even talking about the bun. Many brands continue to use Poor Food ingredients, including high frutose corn syrup (HFCS), MSG, preservatives, fillers, chemical flavorings, modified food starch, and synthetic nitrites. Remember, it isn't the natural nitrites from celery or sea salts that we are trying to avoid—it's the synthetic ones, which may contain lead and arsenic. (See Chapter 2.)

Even companies that work hard to create healthy products can sometimes fall short. Under numerous confusing names, many companies add sugar to enhance the taste of their packaged pooches. While organic sugars may be a step up from HFCS, we still prefer they be left out.

Organic Prairie Organic Uncured Beef Hot Dogs

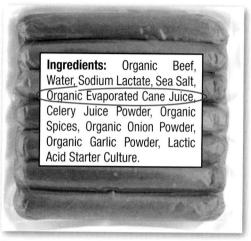

Ingredients: Organic Beef, Water, Sodium Lactate, Sea Salt, Organic Evaporated Cane Juice, Celery Juice Powder, Organic Spices, Organic Onion Powder, Organic Garlic Powder, Lactic Acid Starter Culture.

Even some companies with good intentions add in Poor Food ingredients.

- - - - - - - - - - - - - - - - - - -

Before You Send the Frank to the Doghouse

TODAY, YOU CAN FIND A TON OF GREAT RICH FOOD hot dogs, whether you are looking for a low-fat or good old-fashioned high-fat hot dog. Oh, and today's options allow

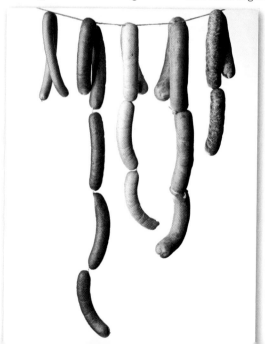

you to expand your taste buds a bit from the traditional beef dog—chicken, turkey, pork, and, yes, even vegan/vegetarian hot dogs are all available.

STEER HERE

OUR TOP PICK! Organic grass-fed hot dogs and organic pasture-raised poultry dogs that are free of additives and sugars.

HOT DOGS BRATS AND SAUSAGE

THE GREATEST ORGANIC ORIGINAL BEEF HOT DOG BY APPLEGATE FARMS

- Grass-fed - Organic - Sugar free - No MSG - No synthetic nitrites
- No artificial flavors/colors

Also try the Greatest Little Organic Uncured Smoky Cocktail Pork Franks, the Great Organic Chicken Hot Dog, and the Great Organic Turkey Hot Dog.

ROCKY MOUNTAIN ORGANIC BEEF HOT DOGS

- Grass-fed - Organic - Sugar free - No MSG - No synthetic nitrites
- No artificial flavors/colors

THE ORIGINAL BRAT HANS ORGANIC SWEET ITALIAN CHICKEN SAUSAGE

- Organic - Sugar free - No MSG - No synthetic nitrites
- No artificial flavors/colors - Five fantastic flavors to enjoy

BILINSKI'S ORGANIC ITALIAN HERB WITH PORCINI MUSHROOMS CHICKEN SAUSAGE

- Organic - Sugar free - No MSG - No synthetic nitrites
- No artificial flavors/colors

AIDELLS ORGANIC SUN DRIED TOMATO SAUSAGE

- Organic - Sugar free - No MSG - No synthetic nitrites
- No artificial flavors/colors

Also try the organic spinach and feta and the sweet basil and roasted garlic.

Note: You may notice that we didn't label our organic choices as free of GMOs, synthetic hormones, and antibiotics. Remember, these facts are true of all organic products. Keep this in mind as we move through the aisles.

STEER CLEAR

HOT DOGS, BRATS, AND SAUSAGE

JENNIE-O TURKEY FRANKS

Contains non-organic mechanically separated turkey, modified food starch, corn syrup solids, dextrose (3 GMOs), sugar (EMD), and sodium nitrite (heavy metal mix-ins). Frankly, Jennie, you could have done much better.

HEBREW NATIONAL DINNER BEEF FRANKS

Contains modified food starch (GMO, gluten), hydrolyzed soy protein (GMO, MSG), synthetic nitrates possibly containing lead and arsenic, and irradiated spices (EMD).

TOFURKY ITALIAN SAUSAGE

This is the best vegan option we could find; it is free of GMOs but still contains wheat gluten, canola oil, and sugar cane.

MEAT

❑ **Choose grass-fed beef hot dogs and brats.**

❑ **Choose organic beef, chicken, pork, or turkey.**

❑ **Choose organic when opting for vegetarian dogs.**

❑ Avoid sugar, cane juice, high fructose corn syrup, and agave syrup.

❑ Avoid MSG.

❑ Avoid preservatives (BHT, BHA, and synthetic nitrates or nitrites).

❑ Avoid antibiotics and hormones.

❑ Avoid artificial flavors or colors.

❑ Avoid GMO ingredients, including soy, corn, canola oil, and tofu.

❑ Avoid added wheat, especially if you are gluten intolerant.

My go-to Rich Food choices for hot dogs, brats, and sausage: _____

_____

_____

_____

_____

_____

_____

_____

_____

_____

_____

_____

_____

_____

Aisle THREE

Fish and Seafood

H ave you heard reports stating that eating greater amounts of fish improves your health? Perhaps you've heard that you should limit your fish intake due to mercury and other toxins. So, which do you believe? Are we healing or hurting ourselves when we have salmon for supper? Should we be serving canned tuna to our tots? Which should we purchase—farmed or wild? Are you drowning in a sea of confusing messaging? No worries. We're here to throw you a line.

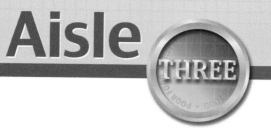

Tipping the Fish Scales

WHEN DECIDING IF A FOOD IS FRIEND OR FOE, we need to weigh two factors—the benefits of the food and the risk involved in eating it. The advantages and the disadvantages of eating fish can be quite hefty. The most obvious reason to eat fish is to obtain the omega-3 polyunsaturated fats found almost exclusively in fish. The essential EPA and DHA found in omega-3 are well documented for their anti-inflammatory benefits, which include a reduction of risk for heart disease, Parkinson's disease, cancer, psoriasis, Alzheimer's disease, and arthritis. Daily intake of DHA has been shown to improve memory by nearly 50 percent within six months. In addition, there is reason to refer to the essential fatty acid omega-3 as the "essential happiness acid," as studies have determined that it is as effective for treating major depression as the prescription drug Prozac. Some fish contain extremely high levels of these otherwise elusive fatty acids, and others contain far less. Eaten by just one out of every three Americans daily, fish offers some big benefits that no other food supplies quite so well.

On the other side of the scale, we have the substantial risk of seafood contamination from by-products of industrial processes, including metals (such as mercury, which affects brain function and development), industrial chemicals (PCBs and dioxins), and pesticides (DDT) that find their way into our waters. These toxins accumulate most in the flesh of the largest predatory fish, like swordfish and shark, who have eaten the greatest majority of toxin-containing smaller fish for the longest period of time. When we eat too much contaminated fish, the mercury, PCBs, dioxins, and pesticides build up in the body and can result in health problems from difficult-to-detect conditions, such as sensory impairment and lack of coordination, to birth defects and cancer.

So, what do we do? Abstain from eating fish to avoid possible toxins, or feast on fish for their essential fatty acids? Many scientists have weighed the pros and cons, and it seems that the benefits outweigh the risks, especially if you choose only the most omega-3 rich fish with the lowest likelihood of toxic exposure. Additionally, recent studies confirm that high levels of the potent antioxidant selenium offer protection from mercury. When selenium in fish comes into contact with mercury, it forms an unbreakable bond. Then, when you eat the fish, the mercury remains bound and unable to cause any damage to your body. So, while the overall risks of smart fish consumption may be minor, we should still strive to choose wisely. Here are seven outstanding seafood selections that are safe from toxins and highly nutritious.

1 Wild Salmon

BASK IN THE BENEFITS: Factory-farmed salmon, which makes up 80 percent of salmon on the global market today, has fewer omega-3s per ounce than wild salmon. Best to whet your appetite with wild varieties like sockeye and coho for more than three times the recommended minimum daily dose of omega-3. Additionally, a Boston University study found that factory-farmed salmon contains only 25 percent of the vitamin D as their free-swimming counterparts. Wild salmon is also an excellent source of the cancer-fighting (and mercury-protective) vitamin selenium.

REDUCE THE RISKS: Farmed salmon are fed fishmeal and receive antibiotics to fight diseases. Tests have shown that farmed salmon contains sixteen times more of the cancer-linked toxin PCB than wild salmon. Artificial colors are often induced in farmed salmon to make them a more appetizing "salmon" pink color, and one of the most commonly used coloring agents, canthaxanthin, has been linked to human eye defects and retinal damage. Choose wild Alaskan salmon for its sustainability and safety.

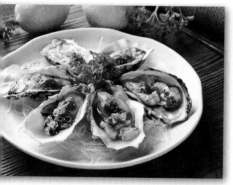

2 Oysters

BASK IN THE BENEFITS: Anchors away for this aphrodisiac! Our pick is Pacific oysters, which are loaded with the autoimmune and libido-boosting essential mineral zinc. These slippery shooters also supply 300 mg of omega-3 per three-ounce serving and nearly 25 percent of the daily requirements for iron.

REDUCE THE RISKS: Farmed oysters account for 95 percent of the world's total oyster consumption, and unlike other fish, farmed mollusks can actually benefit the surrounding coastal waters. Both Pacific oysters and farmed oysters are good options, but steer clear of oysters caught in the Gulf of Mexico, which may have unusually high levels of cadmium due to the 2010 BP oil spill.

3 Wild Rainbow Trout

BASK IN THE BENEFITS: One fish fillet supplies more than 100 percent of the reference daily intake (RDI) for vitamin B12, twice the amount of blood-pressure-lowering potassium contained in a large banana, and nearly half of the RDI for niacin. Niacin is a key micronutrient for metabolism and also offers cholesterol-lowering benefits. This colorful sea creature even surpasses salmon in supplying omega-3.

REDUCE THE RISKS: Lake trout can be tricky. Those caught in Lake Michigan should be avoided due to high levels of toxins while those from Lake Superior are, well . . . superior . . . and are safe to enjoy.

4 Alaskan King Crab

BASK IN THE BENEFITS: These crustaceans deserve the crown for delivering nearly three times your daily requirements for B12 and nearly 70 percent the RDI of your mojo-making mineral zinc—and in only one crab leg. You can also smile because their high levels of omega-3 can lift even the crabbiest person's depression.

REDUCE THE RISKS: Alaskan crab presents virtually no mercury risk. Other great crab suggestions include Dungeness, Kona crab, and Florida stone. These varieties of crab are caught in traps or nets, allowing the release of those not yet to size.

5 Catfish

BASK IN THE BENEFITS: While catfish may only supply moderate levels of omega-3, this whiskered one is just bursting with other benefits. Choose catfish for more than half of your B12 and nearly 200 percent of the bone-building, cancer-fighting, and weight-loss-boosting vitamin D.

REDUCE THE RISKS: While you may not love their unique appearance, you should be enamored with nearly mercury-free filets. Avoid farmed catfish from Southeast Asia, where the use of antibiotics is common.

6 Sardines

BASK IN THE BENEFITS: Small but mighty, sardines supply a huge amount of omega-3s and are loaded with calcium. Fresh or canned, they are a great source of iron, magnesium, phosphorus, potassium, zinc, copper, and manganese. In addition, these silvery, sleek fish are one of the few foods to supply appreciable levels of heart-healthy CoQ10.

REDUCE THE RISKS: Don't turn up your nose at these canned fish; all brands of these nutritional power houses are virtually mercury free.

7 Haddock (aka Scrod)

BASK IN THE BENEFITS: Helping yourself to haddock ensures you two-thirds of your selenium and more than half of your required B12. Try it when making homemade fish and chips.

REDUCE THE RISKS: Purchase line-caught haddock to get the smaller, younger fish that have had less exposure to toxins.

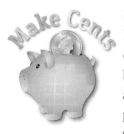

Do you love rainbow trout but live far from Lake Superior? Dying for Maine lobster, but live in California? Frozen seafood may be a great option for you. Many seafood selections are now flash frozen on the boat, just minutes after being caught, which locks in flavor and guarantees high micronutrient content. If fresh, local fish isn't an option, perhaps you should fancy the frozen options. Look for frozen lobster tails, crab legs, shrimp, and fillets when local and fresh is not available. You can save yourself a few clams, because frozen wild seafood costs substantially less than fresh fish.

Seafood Switcheroo

HERE ARE SOME SWIMMERS to swap out of your diet.

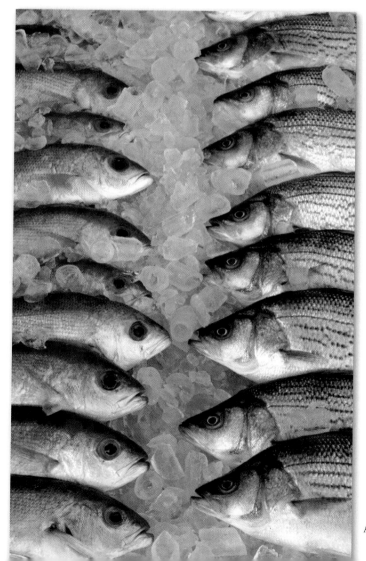

1 Bluefin Tuna

Skip this overfished option with levels of PCBs so high as to warrant warnings. Switch to another steak-like fish, such as line-caught Pacific albacore tuna or Atlantic mackerel.

2 Chilean Sea Bass (aka Patagonian Toothfish)

Oust this over-farmed, buttery sea dweller. This South American catch is high in mercury due to its long life. Switch to catfish for a safer, more sustainable mild-flavored white fish. (We further discuss the importance of sustainability later in this chapter.)

FISH AND SEAFOOD

3 Orange Roughy

This old man of the sea can live to be over one hundred, which gives it a lot of time to absorb mercury and other toxins. Switch to line-caught haddock for a similar taste in recipes.

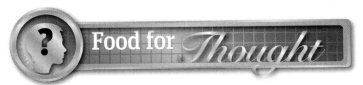

Just as we have farmed land animals for thousands of years, mankind has also dabbled in farming fish. More than two thousand years ago, carp was raised as a second "crop" by Chinese rice farmers right in their rice ponds. Egyptian tombs show carvings of men harvesting tilapia from ponds, and ancient Romans raised fish called *piscinae* in artificial ponds as a status symbol as well as for food and commercial sale. These "farmed" fish, however, were eaten by a very small percentage of people, and the vast majority of the seafood the world population ate was wild.

Today, more than 40 percent of the seafood we eat globally is farmed, and for Americans, that number is closer to 50 percent. With both numbers predicted to climb, are we making the same mistakes with our *aquaculture* as we have with our land-based *agriculture*? The very same concerns we are trying to clean up within land-based factory farms, like overcrowding, unnatural feed and environments, and genetic engineering, are occurring in factory fish farms around the globe.

Aquaculture, like its agriculture equivalent, results in a nutritional loss for us all, supplying fish with fewer of the essential micronutrients. In addition, the environmental costs are great. Scotland's salmon farms, for example, are estimated to produce the same amount of nitrogen waste as the untreated sewage of 3.2 million people—just over half the country's population. Experts also warn that escaped fish have the potential to transmit disease to the wild fish native to our oceans. In Norway alone, nearly half a million farmed salmon and sea trout escape each year and interbreed with wild fish in the North Atlantic. This alters the genetic profile of the wild salmon population and compromises their health. In fact, by 1996, as many as 40 percent of the Atlantic salmon caught in the North Atlantic were of farmed origin.

So why farm fish at all? Some say it is a critical way to hedge against potential shortages and seasonal variations in the harvest of both wild fish and land-sourced meats, but this logic is flawed. It turns out that popular carnivorous species like salmon and shrimp consume several times their weight in fish-derived feed as they produce in edible seafood. Tuna generally requires 20 kilograms of feed to produce just 1 kilogram of tuna. This explains why companies such as Aqua Bounty Technologies are seeking FDA approval for their genetically modified AquAdvantage brand salmon, which will grow year-round and reach market size twice as fast as conventional salmon. Just a little genetic modification and problem solved, right? Or are we opening Pandora's Box?

If we continue to allow genetic engineering of our fish, there could come a day when all of the fish in the ocean are exposed and affected by these genetic mutations (much like today's wheat that you will be introduced to in Chapter 6: Grains).

We urge you to support companies supplying sustainable, wild-caught fish and make its purchase as important as finding organic grass-fed and grass-finished beef and dairy or organic pastured poultry, pork, and eggs. Say no to factory-farmed fish (who eat GMO pellets) and a future of FDA-approved genetically modified fish.

If we are going to farm seafood, perhaps aquaculture would be better off focusing on sedentary mollusks like mussels, oysters, clams, and scallops and leaving the real swimmers alone to roam their natural habitat. These restaurant favorites don't eat GMO-based feed pellets or deplete the small fish populations. Done correctly, sustainable mollusk aquaculture can be one of the most environmentally friendly types of aquaculture—helping with filtration and nitrogen removal in the surrounding wild waters. Plus, there is little chance these little guys will escape.

• • • • • • • • • • • • • • •

There Are Only So Many Fish in the Sea—
Understanding Sustainability

DUE TO RADICAL FISHING PRACTICES that exploit fish stocks and destroy the marine environment, the ability and likelihood of certain fish to breed, survive, and thrive is being threatened. In other words, their sustainability is in question, and not only is the future of fish a huge question mark, so is the health of future generations who will not benefit from the healthy advantages (and great taste) of consuming fish.

Bluefin tuna occupies most of the northern Atlantic Ocean and is perhaps the most popular endangered fish of the nearly 150 species of fish on the endangered list. One of the fastest fish in the sea, they can grow to 10 feet in length and weigh in at nearly 1,400 pounds. This fish's reputation as a tough catch has made it highly prized among sport fishermen, and as a consequence, is heavily overfished. Most marine experts agree that without regulation and intervention, they will become extinct.

If we are not going to purchase factory-farmed fish, what are we to do? How do we ensure that the wild-caught fish we are buying is being caught in a responsible, *sustainable* way? One option is to buy fish that is part of a sustainable fishing program like the Marine Stewardship Council (MSC)—a nonprofit global certification program that uses impartial third-party verification. Look for the blue MSC ecolabel to ensure wild-caught sustainability, so your favorite fish can be enjoyed for years to come.

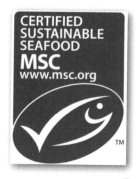

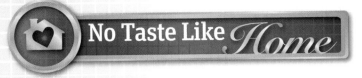
No Taste Like *Home*

Fish sticks may sound like a good option for your little ones, but beware.
Most store-bought brands are made with farmed fish and are loaded with unwanted Poor Food
ingredients like wheat, modified starches, and canola oil.

Swimmingly Good Fish Sticks

INGREDIENTS

- 1 pound wild white fish (can be frozen and thawed)
- 2 large pastured eggs, whisked
- 1 cup organic almond flour (or grind your own soaked almonds to powder)
- 1 tsp. unrefined sea salt
- Coconut oil for frying

DIRECTIONS

1 Clean and pat dry fish.

2 Cut fish into strips (approximately 1-inch wide and 6-inches long). Remove bones as you cut.

3 Beat eggs in a small bowl and place the almond flour mixed with the salt onto a plate.

4 Heat oil.

5 Coat each fish strip with egg wash and dip both sides in almond flour. Place on a clean plate until the oil is hot.

6 Fry both sides of strips until brown and crispy.

7 Serve with homemade ketchup or tartar sauce (see page 152) or with organic vinegar.

STEER HERE

- Wild, fatty, cold-water fish: Alaskan salmon, anchovies, herring, sardines
- Wild rainbow trout (Lake Superior preferred)
- Wild, small-line-caught albacore tuna
- Line-caught haddock
- Atlantic mackerel
- Alaskan King, Dungeness, Kona, and Florida stone crab
- Wild catfish
- Wild-caught spiny lobster
- Mussels
- Pacific oysters
- Squid

FISH

MARKET PANTRY FROZEN ALASKAN KETA SALMON

● Wild caught ● Frozen ● Omega-3 ● MSC Certified

STEER CLEAR

FISH

GORTON'S CLASSIC FISH STICKS

This classic is no catch! The fish is minced. That's right—you are eating fish scraps coated in wheat flour (gluten belly—see page 175), canola or soybean oil (GMO), corn flour (GMO), dextrose (GMO sugar), sugar (EMD), and caramel color (possible carcinogen). And what do the next six ingredients—modified corn starch, hydrolyzed corn gluten, monosodium glutamate, autolyzed yeast extract, disodium inosinate, disodium guanylate—have in common? They're all aliases for MSG. That is a lot of obesity-inducing flavor enhancer in an itsy-bitsy fish stick.

- Farmed salmon
- Bluefin tuna
- Swordfish
- Shark
- Orange roughy

- Marlin
- Chilean sea bass
- Any fish , farmed or wild, imported from Asia (polluted waters, poor chemical regulation)

FISH AND SEAFOOD

☐ Choose wild over farmed fish.

☐ Choose fatty cold-water fish for high omega-3.

☐ Choose line-caught (label may read troll caught or hook-and-line caught) fish.

☐ Choose farmed mollusks. They are fair game.

☐ Avoid the larger predatory fish to reduce mercury intake.

☐ Avoid farmed salmon—always!

☐ Avoid eating species that are over-farmed.

Checkout Checklist

*My go-to Rich Food choices for fish and seafood:*_____

_____

Packaged Fish

CANNED TUNA AND SALMON are convenient, tasty, and versatile. There are some ways to ensure that there isn't anything fishy about your canned options.

Tuna

Many people enjoy tuna grilled over an open fire, served as sashimi or sushi, or from a can. There are, however, three things you need to know in order to purchase the safest, most micronutrient-rich tuna: the type of tuna, how the tuna is caught, and how it is packaged.

Wild-caught tuna is ultimately what you are looking for, but choose only those labeled troll-caught or pole-caught to ensure younger, smaller-sized fish, with less time exposed to possible contaminants. Pole-caught fish are typically in better, tastier condition than their mass-caught rivals because they do not get battered and bruised in nets, nor do they die at sea hours before returning to port, as does tuna caught with long lines (a method of deep water, unsustainable fishing that should be avoided).

Next, you will have to decide which type of canned tuna to put in your cart: white or light, which has slightly darker shading than white tuna. For light tuna, favor tongol or skipjack over bluefin or yellowfin for sustainability and lower contaminant levels. Albacore, on the other hand, is the only species of tuna that can be sold as white in the United States. When *Consumer Reports* tested mercury levels in canned tuna, they found vastly different contamination levels. The light tuna sample with the most mercury still had less than the white tuna sample with the least mercury. You can see how important choosing light tuna can be if you are concerned about mercury levels. However, many great companies are fishing only the small white albacore. This reduces the mercury levels in the albacore to levels similar to light tuna and contains nearly twice the omega-3 as their light counterparts. You can be assured our Rich Food options are amongst these standouts!

Finally, we need to consider how the tuna is packaged. When buying canned tuna, it is important to choose either solid-packed tuna (packed without any added liquid) or tuna packed in water over oil for two reasons. First, the oil used is often high in omega-6 (think inflammation), the type of fat that we are trying to balance with the anti-inflammatory omega-3. Second, the oil pulls out many of the fat-soluble vitamins and omega-3 when we drain and rinse the tuna. Both the solid and water-packed eliminate these issues.

Now that we've discovered what liquid is nutritionally best for packaging, let's examine the material used in packaging. As you might remember in our discussion of label losers in Chapter 2, we must be mindful of bisphenol-A, or BPA, in our canned food. Lining some cans, BPA has been linked to a variety of disorders, including cancer, obesity, and reproductive disorders. Support brands that clearly label their cans BPA free, purchase fillets in glass jars, or attempt to purchase tuna in BPA-free pouches. Remember, as we stated earlier, not all manufacturers are labeling their BPA-free cans clearly, but be assured that all the products in our Steer Here section are free of this Poor Food perpetrator.

Smoked Salmon

Smoked salmon is salmon that is salted and smoked at high temperatures to keep it edible for an extended period of time. Today, most of us associate smoked salmon with bagels and cream cheese, but there are many other ways to enjoy this healthy, micronutrient-packed food. Try smoked salmon in an omelet, over a salad, as a pizza topping, in tarts and quiches, or as a colorful appetizer at your next dinner party. Be careful when choosing a smoked salmon—most are farmed and contain added sugars, colors, and preservatives.

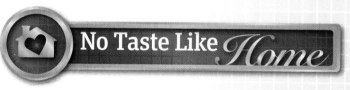

Party Perfect Pinwheels

INGREDIENTS
- 8 ounces softened cream cheese (see page 78 for our Rich Food choices)
- 1 Tbsp. fresh lemon juice
- 8 ounces sliced wild caught smoked salmon
- ¼ tsp. unrefined salt
- $1/_8$ tsp. organic white pepper

DIRECTIONS

 1 Add your choice of chopped dill, diced jalapenos, diced arugula (all organic).

 2 Lay salmon slices side by side on a flat sheet, slightly overlapping to form a rectangle.

 3 Combine all ingredients and any other desired seasonings in a bowl and mix until smooth.

 4 Spread mixture evenly across salmon.

 5 Slowly and tightly roll salmon. You should be left with a tubular salmon-like stick.

 6 Cut salmon tubes in 1-inch increments. (Cut diagonally for an impressive presentation.)

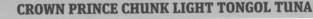

STEER HERE

LIGHT TUNA

CROWN PRINCE CHUNK LIGHT TONGOL TUNA

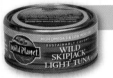

- Wild caught • Water packed • BPA free • Low mercury
- Omega-3 • No salt added • Dolphin safe certified

Pull-top lids make these great to-go snacks!

NATURAL SEA LIGHT YELLOW FIN TUNA AND TONGOL TUNA

- Wild caught • Water packed • BPA free • Low mercury
- Omega-3 • No salt added • Dolphin safe

WILD PLANET WILD SKIPJACK LIGHT TUNA

- Pole-or line-caught • Wild caught • Water packed
- BPA free (you won't see this on the label, but we asked)
- Low mercury • Omega-3 • Dolphin safe

WHITE TUNA

AMERICAN TUNA

- Pole caught • Wild caught • Solid packed • BPA free
- No salt added • Low to moderate mercury • High in omega-3
- MSC certified sustainable • Dolphin safe

These hand-packed sashimi-grade albacore loins are pole caught by six fishing families and contain an incredible 8,000 to 10,000 mg of omega-3 per six-ounce serving. It is canned with organic jalapenos or garlic.

VITAL CHOICE CANNED NATURAL PACK ALBACORE TUNA

- Pole caught • Wild caught • Solid packed—no draining • BPA free
- No salt added • Low to moderate mercury • High in omega-3
- MSC certified sustainable • Dolphin safe

SALMON

NATURAL SEA CANNED RED SOCKEYE SALMON NO SALT ADDED

- Pole caught
- Wild caught
- Solid packed—no draining
- BPA free
- No salt added
- Very low mercury
- Moderate omega-3
- MSC certified sustainable
- Dolphin safe

VITAL CHOICE WILD RED CANNED SOCKEYE SALMON

- Pole caught
- Wild caught
- Solid packed
- BPA free
- No salt added
- Very low mercury
- Moderate omega-3
- MSC certified sustainable
- Dolphin safe
- Contains the skin and edible bones, which adds essential micronutrients

VITAL CHOICE SOCKEYE SALMON NOVA LOX

- Pole caught
- Wild caught
- Free of sugar and artificial colors
- MSC certified sustainable

ECHO FALLS WILD ALASKAN SOCKEYE SMOKED SALMON

- Wild caught
- Free of sugar and artificial colors

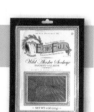

STEER CLEAR

TUNA

BUMBLE BEE LUNCH ON THE RUN TUNA SALAD

Run away now! Sixty-eight ingredients make up this catastrophe filled with GMOs, sweeteners, EMDs, emulsifiers, and trans fats. The sugar, which appears in the tuna salad, crackers, cookie, and peaches that comprise this lunch, totals a whopping 30 grams—that's more sugar than a Butterfinger candy bar.

FISH AND SEAFOOD

STARKIST TUNA SWEET & SPICY CHUNK LIGHT
(IN OIL WITH PEPPERS)

This is part of the Starkist Authentico line of flavored tunas, but this sweet and spicy number may contain a lot more than you bargained for. It comes in a BPA-lined can, is packaged in oil that leaches out fat-soluble vitamins and omega-3 from the tuna, and contains sugar (EMD), corn syrup (EMD, GMO), soybean oil (GMO), soy flour (GMO), autolyzed yeast extract (MSG), and phosphoric acid (another one of our EMD enemies).

SMOKED SALMON

NATHAN'S NOVA SALMON (CLASSIC SMOKED)

Like most other store-bought farmed salmon, this nova contains corn syrup and corn or soy oil (all GMO). And don't be fooled by its lovely salmon shade—five artificial coloring chameleons appear on the ingredient list.

☐ Choose wild-caught tuna or salmon, preferably troll-, pole-, or line-caught.

☐ Choose tongol or skipjack as your "light" options.

☐ Choose smaller pole-caught albacore as your "white" option.

☐ Choose water packed or solid packed to avoid micronutrient loss.

☐ Choose BPA-free cans, glass jars, or pouches.

☐ Choose Marine Stewardship Council (MSC) Certified sustainable products where available.

☐ Choose salmon salad as a nutritious alternative to tuna salad.

☐ Avoid high-toxin bluefin and yellowfin tuna.

☐ Avoid added ingredients, including sugars and refined salts.

☐ Avoid artificial colors.

*My go-to Rich Food choices for packaged fish:*_____

_____

Aisle FOUR

Produce

Produce is the last stop on our grocery store perimeter tour. A stroll through the produce department, with its brightly colored fruits and vegetables and intermittent misting showers, can feel like a walk through a real farmers market, complete with wooden crates and handwritten signs. Unfortunately, an uninformed shopper can easily be duped in this department.

Of the vast variety of vegetables and fantastic fruits offered, how can we identify the Rich Food pick of the crop? The first step in finding any Rich Food, as mentioned earlier, is to locate those that have the highest micronutrient values with minimal losses from Poor Food storage and shipping methods. Then, we must choose the foods that have the lowest risk of causing us harm (i.e., contain pesticides, carcinogens, GMOs, and so on). Let's examine how we can accomplish these two things in the produce department.

The Hunt for High Micronutrient Values

FINDING THE MOST micronutrient-rich fruits and vegetables is easy. The rule of thumb is to pick fruits and vegetables that have been grown locally, which is defined as foods grown or raised within a one-hundred-mile radius. Why? Well, every minute of every mile that your food travels matters, because as fresh food is exposed to environmental elements—heat, light, and oxygen—it loses precious micronutrients.

To reach your goal of micronutrient sufficiency, you should strive to eat the most freshly picked produce possible. For most of us, the thought of sitting down to a meal filled with produce picked just moments before is little more than a pipe dream. However, this was not always the case.

"In 1945, 40 percent of all vegetables consumed in the United States were grown in back-yards," says Joel Salatin, author of *Folks, This Ain't Normal: A Farmer's Advice for Happier Hens, Healthier People, and a Better World.* However, the Leopold Center for Sustainable Agriculture at Iowa State University reports that these days, the average potato has traveled 1,155 miles before it reaches your dinner table. Similarly, a tomato travels 1,569 miles, and a carrot travels an exhaust-ing, micronutrient-depleting 1,838 miles prior to being served!

So, how does this distance really affect the micronutrients in the produce we purchase? To an-swer this question, we turn to research conducted at Penn State University on spinach's ability to retain micronutrients. The study showed that when stored at a cool 68 degrees Fahrenheit, it only took four days for spinach to lose 47 percent of its folate (vitamin B9) and carotenoid content. Even in moderate ambient temperatures, the back of a container truck can get much hotter than 68 de-grees Fahrenheit (20 degrees Celsius), and the hotter it is, the faster micronutrient loss occurs. The Penn State researchers found that even when the spinach was kept in a refrigerator at 39 degrees Fahrenheit (4 degrees Celsius), perhaps similar to your local grocery store or restaurant cooler, it lost an average of 53 percent of its folate and carotenoid content in ap-proximately one week.

Another advantage to buying local produce is that it often has more micronutrients to begin with. This is because local farmers allow their produce to fully ripen prior to bringing it to market. Most large-scale conventional farming opera-tions are essentially forced to harvest produce early, prior to its reaching peak ripeness, in order for it to withstand mechanical harvesting and long-distance travel without damage or spoilage. This premature picking is detrimen-tal to a food's overall micronutrient value.

According to Harvard Medical School's Center for Health and the Global Environment, full color may be achieved after harvest, while nutritional quality may not. Tomatoes, for example, will increase in vitamin C after being prematurely harvested; however, they will never reach the micronutrient levels of those that ripen on the vine. This is particularly important with tomatoes as they make up one-quarter of Americans' total vegetable consumption.

Ditch the Potential Dangers

OKAY, SO LOCAL PRODUCE IS BEST at supplying the most micronutrients, but how about the second half of the Rich Food equation? How can we identify produce that won't cause harm to our bodies? What kind of potential harm are we talking about, and how great is the risk to us in the first place? The dangers that we can encounter in the produce aisle come from two distinct sources: GMOs and pesticide residue. In Chapter 2, we explained why GMOs should be avoided and how prevalent they are in your grocery store. The good news is that while the vast majority of the boxed and brightly packaged foods in other departments contain GMOs in one form or another, in the produce department, there are only four fruits and vegetables that are genetically modified: zucchini, crookneck (yellow) squash, Hawaiian papaya, and sweet corn (white and yellow varieties). While potatoes and tomatoes were once genetically modified, smart consumers boycotted these problematic produce. Recently, apples have been genetically modified to prevent them from turning brown when spoiling. Grocery giants haven't yet made their decision on whether or not to carry these un-browning beauties. However, we hope consumers will take a stand again and not purchase them. After all, who wants to eat a rotten apple, even if it doesn't look it?

While we may only have four foods on our GMO produce watch list, the number gets considerably longer when we take into account pesticide residue. Over four hundred chemical pesticides are routinely used in conventional farming, many of which are known to cause cancer and lead to problems of the nervous and endocrine systems. Children are especially vulnerable due to their smaller body size and immature nervous and endocrine systems. In fact, the average child may receive as much as four times more exposure to at least eight widely used cancer-causing pesticides than an adult. By avoiding foods that may be genetically modified or are known to contain high levels of chemical pesticide residue, you can safeguard your family against unnecessary exposure in the produce department. The good news is that the answer comes down to two little words you are already familiar with: *buy organic!*

Breaking the PLU Code

WOULDN'T IT BE NICE IF PRODUCE WERE LABELED so that we could differentiate an organic apple from a conventional apple, or a genetically modified zucchini from an organic zucchini? The fruit or vegetable may not look different or smell different, but many times, you will find a PLU sticker—short for "price lookup codes"—affixed to your grocery store produce. Those pesky stickers may be a pain to remove sometimes, but what they tell you can help keep you and your family out of harm's way.

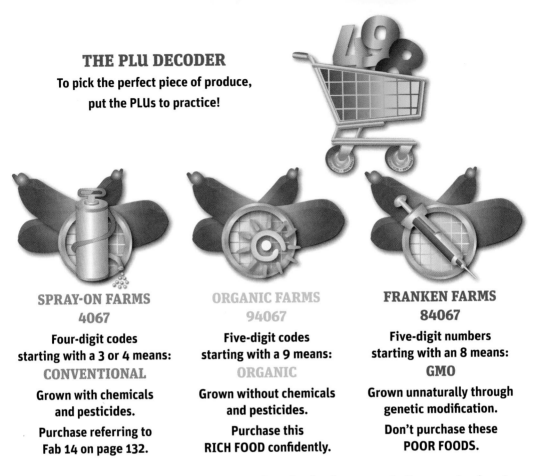

THE PLU DECODER
To pick the perfect piece of produce, put the PLUs to practice!

SPRAY-ON FARMS
4067

Four-digit codes
starting with a 3 or 4 means:
CONVENTIONAL

Grown with chemicals
and pesticides.

Purchase referring to
Fab 14 on page 132.

ORGANIC FARMS
94067

Five-digit codes
starting with a 9 means:
ORGANIC

Grown without chemicals
and pesticides.

Purchase this
RICH FOOD confidently.

FRANKEN FARMS
84067

Five-digit numbers
starting with an 8 means:
GMO

Grown unnaturally through
genetic modification.

Don't purchase these
POOR FOODS.

Be a stickler for the sticker. Try to locate produce that has been organically grown by choosing those PLUs that start with the number 9 as well as looking for organic signs in the produce section. This guarantees that you are not eating genetically modified food or adding to your body's toxic load and that your selection offers maximum micronutrient value.

Can you see the problem with this yet? Many fruits and vegetables don't have stickers on them. And even if they did, no government agency yet mandates that GMO foods be properly and clearly labeled. Even the biggest proponent of GMO seeds admits consumer awareness would be an industry killer:

"If you put a label on genetically engineered food you might as well put a skull and crossbones on it."
—NORMAN BRAKSICK, president of Asgrow Seed Company, a subsidiary of Monsanto (the largest proponent of GMO seeds)

Because GMO producers realize that their produce would be picked over, you will very rarely see one labeled with a five-digit PLU code beginning with an 8. Hopefully in the near future, however, this voluntary labeling may become law and all produce will be required to carry these important PLU stickers, indicating to consumers how their food has been grown.

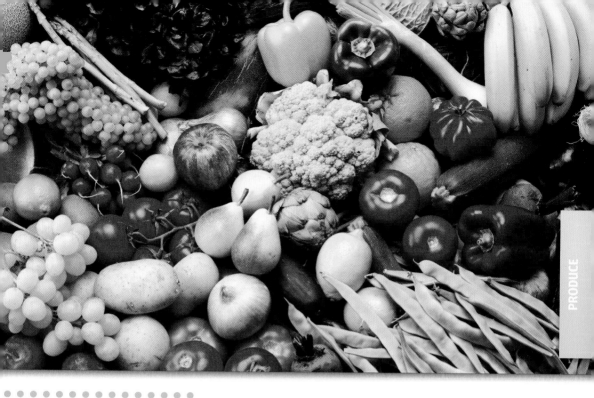

The Fab Fourteen and Terrible Twenty

SO, WHAT SHOULD YOU DO? Obviously, the proponents of GMOs aren't going to help us avoid their produce. In a perfect world, the best option to protect you from all harm would be to only purchase organic produce. But who said life is perfect? This is the real world—where we pay real bills and have real budgets. We have to make choices on where to spend our grocery money. To help make this decision easier, we offer you our very own Rich Food, Poor Food produce list to convey which fruits and vegetables are safe to buy conventionally (the Fab Fourteen) and which ones you should never buy conventionally (the Terrible Twenty).

In creating our list, we first took the Environmental Working Group's yearly compilation of the cleanest and dirtiest produce in terms of pesticide residue. This protected us from toxins but didn't take into account GMOs. So, next we asked Jeffrey Smith, executive director of the Institute for Responsible Technology, for his recommendations on how to best avoid GMO produce.

By utilizing this easy-to-use produce guide, you can reduce your pesticide exposure by 80 percent and avoid GMO produce 100 percent of the time! If you cannot find a particular fruit or vegetable on the list, that means it fell in the middle somewhere or was not ranked. In these cases, use your best judgment. If you can get it organic without paying too much more, do so; if not, buy it conventionally.

Photocopy page 132, or download your free wallet-size version of the following list from the Calton Nutrition Rich Food Resource Center online and bring it with you to the grocery store to pick safe produce that doesn't break the bank.

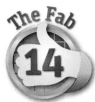

The Fab 14

Purchase these conventionally with little risk of GMO or pesticide residue.

1 Onions
2 Pineapples
3 Avocado
4 Cabbage
5 Sweet peas (frozen)
6 Asparagus
7 Mangoes
8 Eggplant
9 Kiwi
10 Cantaloupe
11 Sweet potatoes
12 Grapefruit
13 Watermelon
14 Mushrooms

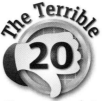

The Terrible 20

Choose organic to reduce the risk of GMO and pesticide residue.

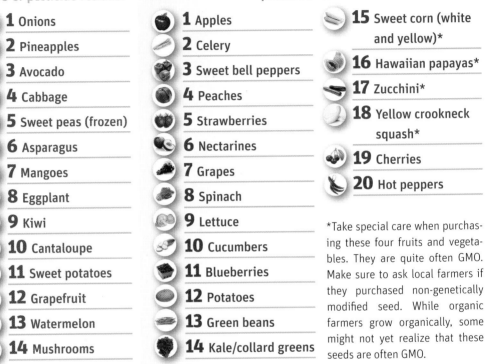

1 Apples
2 Celery
3 Sweet bell peppers
4 Peaches
5 Strawberries
6 Nectarines
7 Grapes
8 Spinach
9 Lettuce
10 Cucumbers
11 Blueberries
12 Potatoes
13 Green beans
14 Kale/collard greens

15 Sweet corn (white and yellow)*
16 Hawaiian papayas*
17 Zucchini*
18 Yellow crookneck squash*
19 Cherries
20 Hot peppers

*Take special care when purchasing these four fruits and vegetables. They are quite often GMO. Make sure to ask local farmers if they purchased non-genetically modified seed. While organic farmers grow organically, some might not yet realize that these seeds are often GMO.

As with the other perimeter aisles we have visited thus far, by purchasing organic produce, you protect yourself from harmful pesticides, GMOs, chemical fertilizers, various synthetic substances, sewage sludge, and irradiation, while making a stand regarding your health, community, and environment.

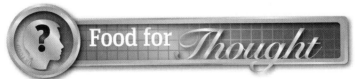

Food for Thought

Have you noticed a lot of seedless fruits and exotic new vegetable varieties in the produce department? These novel products result from natural, selective breeding and not genetic engineering. So go ahead—it's safe to enjoy those seedless grapes, crossbred broccoflower (broccoli and cauliflower), and hybrid plumcots (plum and apricot). After all, variety is the spice of life.

A Masterpiece of Colors

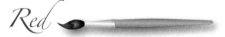

WE NOW HAVE A PLAN for purchasing our produce. But with so many outstanding varieties of fruits and vegetables available to us, how should we choose which ones to serve in our salads or steam for our side dishes? Just like a painter must have a variety of possible paint colors to choose from when creating his masterpiece, you too will benefit from choosing produce from the broadest range of colors.

Think of optimal health as the finest masterpiece you can paint. In order to create it, you will need to consume foods of many different colors. As it so happens, a fruit or vegetable's color can tell you a lot about what micronutrients it will deliver. The color of the skin is determined by the specific plant compounds it contains, and those in the same color family will deliver similar nutrients and health benefits. Your job is to add a bit of each color to your daily dietary color palette so that you can obtain an ideal range of micronutrients every day and paint your way to optimal health.

Red

From crimson and cardinal to ruby and rose, there are two antioxidants, lycopene and anthocyanin, responsible for the red color in produce. The first, lycopene, is a powerful antioxidant associated with reduced incidence of cancer, cardiovascular disease, and macular degeneration. It is also said to lower LDL (the so-called bad cholesterol), enhance the body's immunity, and protect enzymes, DNA, and cellular fats from free radical damage. Lycopene is also great for athletes, as it may help with shortness of breath and exercise-induced asthma. Anthocyanin, which is richly concentrated in the pigments of berries, has been shown to possibly aid in pain relief, depression, and anxiety.

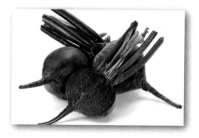

LIFT YOUR MOOD. The lycopene in tomatoes can help lift depression by reducing inflammation. The iron and vitamin B6 in tomatoes also work together to create mood-regulating neurotransmitters such as dopamine, serotonin, and norepinephrine. Additionally, the magnesium in tomatoes works as a mild mood tranquilizer that regulates energy levels and reduces stress.

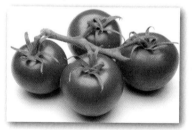

BOOST YOUR ENDURANCE. No one will *beet* you in the race when you add these red beauties into your diet. Researchers from Exeter University in England discovered that beets helped athletes increase their endurance by up to 16 percent. The beets allowed cyclists' muscles to tolerate high-intensity exercise longer by reducing the amount of oxygen used during exercise.

PRODUCE

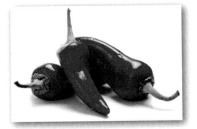

FIRE UP YOUR DIET. Ignite your diet by adding some hot red peppers to your breakfast. According to a study in the *British Journal of Nutrition,* adding capsaicin, the compound that gives peppers their heat, to your morning meal will decrease your hunger throughout the day by moderating levels of the "hunger hormone" ghrelin. But don't worry about getting too fired up—your brain is filled with receptors for capsaicin. When triggered, they release endorphins that calm you down naturally.

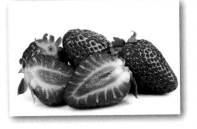

YOU'LL BE BERRY, BERRY BEAUTIFUL. Who doesn't want younger-looking skin? Strawberries are an excellent source of both ellagic acid and vitamin C, which help protect skin from environmental damage. Ellagic acid aids in your skin's ability to retain moisture and may also reduce age spots, while vitamin C is essential for collagen. Maintaining optimal dietary vitamin C levels has been associated with fewer wrinkles and, yes, younger-looking skin.

Looking to whiten that smile? Eating berries may do the trick. Strawberries contain salicylic acid, a natural tooth whitener often found in tooth care products.

Orange

Orange foods are orange because of their high levels of a micronutrient known as beta-carotene. As the orange member of a family of plant pigments called carotenoids, beta-carotene is most often associated with oranges (as we would expect), winter squash, sweet potatoes, carrots, pumpkins, mangoes, and cantaloupe, to name a few. Beta-carotene is also known as pro-vitamin A, because it can convert to vitamin A (retinal) once inside your body. However, a recent study conducted by Johns Hopkins Bloomberg School of Public Health and published in the *Journal of Nutrition* found that the rate of this conversion is likely near 21 to 1. So if you are looking for the cancer-fighting, anti-viral, eyesight-improving benefits of vitamin A, you will want to eat a lot of beta-carotene! But remember, sometimes the brightly colored skin of citrus fruits can be deceiving. Oranges are often colored with counterfeit colors to make them appear more appetizing (see page 23 for more details).

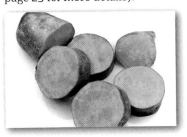

MAXIMIZE MUSCLE PERFORMANCE. Beta-carotene is only one of the micronutrient superstars in sweet potatoes. As it turns out, sweet potatoes contain even more potassium than a banana, and their higher fiber content prevents the spikes in blood sugar that happen when you eat regular spuds. Extra potassium can be especially important to fitness buffs because sufficient amounts help ensure proper muscle function and prevent muscle cramps.

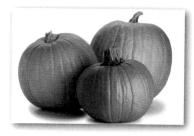

THINK LIKE A GENIUS. Pumpkins are true brain boosters. Pumpkins are great sources of beta-cryptoxanthin, a carotenoid cousin to beta-carotene that has been shown to improve learning ability and fend off cognitive decline. Pumpkin seeds are also high in zinc, which has been shown to improve memory, reasoning, and hand-eye coordination. Maybe the "Headless Horseman" was as smart as he was scary.

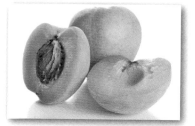

FLUSH THE FAT. Have you always wanted to eat your way to thin? According to a study in the *British Journal of Nutrition,* the carotenoids in apricots improve the body's ability to detoxify the liver, which in turn enhances fat metabolism. So when you put it all together, perhaps an apricot a day can help to keep the pounds at bay.

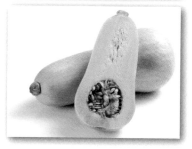

SQUASH HEALTH PROBLEMS BEFORE THEY HAPPEN. Not only does warm winter squash taste amazing, it is (like all orange foods on this list) bursting with carotenoids. Research has determined that individuals who eat a diet high in carotenoid-rich vegetables were 43 percent less likely to develop age-related macular degeneration (AMD)—a common eye disorder which can lead to blindness. What's more, men were 36 percent less likely to die of a heart attack.

Yellow

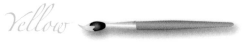

Yellow foods are touted for their high levels of beta-cryptoxanthin, the brain-booster we discussed in the pumpkin comments. Eat and get smarter with yellow squash, yellow bell pepper, pineapples, grapefruits, and yellow sweet corn.

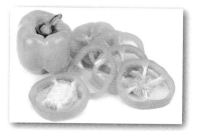

BURN FAT, BOOST ENERGY. When you think of vitamin C, you think oranges, right? Well, the truth is, yellow bell peppers have nearly five and a half times more (341 mg vs. 63 mg) vitamin C content per serving than a serving of oranges. When Arizona State University looked at people who supplemented vitamin C, they found that they burned more fat than those who were deficient. What most people don't know is that your body needs vitamin C to synthesize carnitine, a compound that exerts a substantial antioxidant action and helps convert fat into energy.

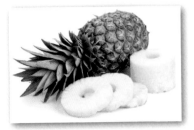

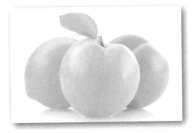

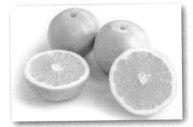

DELIGHTFUL DIGESTION. The core of the pineapple contains an enzyme called bromelain, which helps you digest your food by breaking down protein. Bromelain also has anti-cancer, anti-inflammatory, and anti-clotting properties. Pineapples are high in the essential mineral manganese, whose name derives from the Greek word *magnesia,* meaning magic. Studies have shown that eating pineapple regularly helps fight against arthritis and indigestion.

TURN BACK TIME. Who even knew yellow plums existed? But they do, and if you see them, grab a few! According to a study in the *Journal of the Neurological Sciences,* yellow plums contain chlorogenic acid, a natural substance proven to fight the oxidative stress that prematurely ages our skin. And if that's not good enough, these plums also contain high amounts of pro-vitamin A, which helps increase skin-cell production to ward off fine lines, and vitamin C, which helps build collagen to keep skin elastic and supple. These yellow plums can create beauty from the inside out!

WEIGHT-LOSS WONDER! While hearing someone talk about going on a grapefruit diet may make you giggle, it turns out that grapefruits have been clinically shown to benefit dieters in two important ways. First, according to a study done at the Nutrition and Metabolic Research Center at Scripps Clinic, there exists a physiological link between grapefruit and insulin. It is speculated that chemical properties in grapefruit reduce insulin levels and encourage weight loss. Second, according to Austrian research, the aroma of a grapefruit stimulates the release of serotonin and activates the body's satiety center in the hypothalamus, making you feel genuinely full without overeating. While some of the grapefruit diets are extreme and thus not recommended by medical experts, including regular servings of grapefruit in your diet offers outstanding health and weight-management benefits.

Green

You may remember from your middle school science class that green plants and vegetables get their green color from a substance called chlorophyll. Chlorophyll has been shown to be antibacterial and stimulate the growth and maintenance of lean muscle tissue. Green foods are also the richest source of the dynamic duo zeaxanthin and lutein (more carotenoids), which have been shown in many studies to reduce the risk of chronic eye diseases, including cataracts and age-related macular degeneration (AMD).

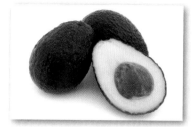

GET YOUR GLOW ON. Here is a fruit that will help you achieve a healthy glow, whether you eat it or use it as a spa mask. Due to its high levels of essential fatty acids that are naturally found in skin cells and help to keep your skin smooth and supple, the avocado is an age-old beauty secret. When topically applied, it has the added ability to stimulate collagen and elastin production. Mix a little avocado with sour cream (which contains lactic acid to help exfoliate dead skin) and apply to your face for about ten minutes before washing it off with water.

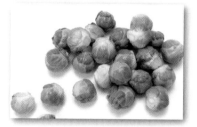

THE LITTLE GREEN FAT-FIGHTING MACHINE. Most people make a face when you mention brussels sprouts, but you may want to give them another try based on new research showing their ability to burn fat. Brussels sprouts contain indole-3-carbinol, which increases production of adiponectin, a hormone that tells your body to burn stored fat for fuel. Think of them as little green fat-burning machines!

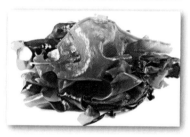

REV UP YOUR METABOLISM. If you are not snacking on seaweed, you don't know what you are missing. When we experience low energy, most of us grab for a sugar and caffeine-filled energy drink or coffee concoction, but did you know it may be iodine that your body is really craving? When we are iodine deficient, the thyroid—which controls metabolism—begins to stall, making you feel sluggish. Kelp is a great source of natural iodine. Try it for a week or two, and watch your energy return. Look for more information on these great, ready-to-eat kelp options in Aisle 8: Snacks.

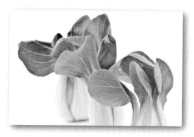

CUT THE SKIN CANCER RISK. That's right, an eleven-year study of 1,360 Australian adults found that those who ate the most leafy green vegetables, like kale, chard, and bok choy, reduced their risk of getting squamous cell carcinoma (the second most common type of skin cancer) by 54 percent compared with those who ate the least. Green leafy vegetables are rich in carotenoids (lutein and zeaxanthin) and a wide variety of other micronutrients that can help guard against UV-induced free-radical damage and may help block tumor development in skin exposed to UV radiation.

Purple and Blue

The rich blue and purple tones in your produce are courtesy of some pretty special flavonoids called anthocyanins. These colorful characters are powerful antioxidants that protect your cells from damage. They may reduce cancer and stroke risks, improve memory, and even aid in longevity. The variety of shades is almost as impressive as the long list of health benefits. You won't have anything to be blue about when your health is improved from enjoying these bold-colored beauties, which include plums, grapes, berries, and eggplant.

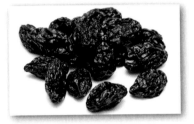

PLUM PERFECT FOR YOUR BONES. Prunes (dried plums) are not only loaded with antioxidants, they contain three essential bone-building micronutrients: boron, potassium, and vitamin K. A Florida State University study suggested that eating a serving of prunes every day stopped bone loss and increased bone density in post-menopausal women. The high fiber content in these wrinkled wonders also reduced hunger in study participants. Osteoporosis is the pits. To reduce your risk for it, enjoy these pitted delights.

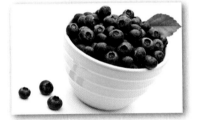

BERRY BOOST. Feeling sluggish in the mid-afternoon? A handful of blueberries should do the trick for a quick energy kick. The phenolics in these mini miracles help moderate insulin and blood sugar, which can keep you even-keeled at that time of day when one out of three women report feeling tired. Also, blueberry's antioxidants increase the blood flow to the brain, improving neuron function to help your mind stay strong.

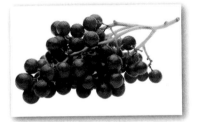

VANISH VARICOSE VEINS. Grapes contain proanthocyanidins, which play a role in the stabilization of collagen and maintenance of elastin. These compounds have been shown to repair and strengthen veins and shrink varicose veins by 41 percent in only two months. Additionally, grape phenolics have been researched for their anti-obesity effect. This means grapes may be your fast track to a younger, leaner you.

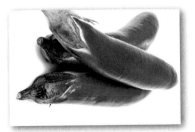

BE VICTORIOUS OVER VIRUSES. Don't let a virus get you down. Fight back with antiviral eggplant. The antiviral activity of the eggplant comes from the chlorogenic acid it contains. Other benefits of this acid, one of the most potent free-radical scavengers in plant tissue, include anticancer, antimicrobial, and anti-LDL ("bad" cholesterol) properties. It's lights out for viruses when you include this purple powerhouse in your diet.

White

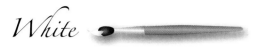

When you think about apples, bananas, and cucumbers, the color white is probably not what jumps to mind. However, it is the white flesh of these fruits and vegetables that brings them to our white painter's palette. Add to that list cauliflower and pears, and you have a set of superstars that can reduce stroke risk by 52 percent! A recent ten-year study concluded that these white-fleshed fruits and vegetables, rich in the flavonoid quercetin, were better than green, orange, yellow, red, or blue/purple fruits and vegetables at reducing the risk of strokes. That apple a day may just keep the doctor away after all!

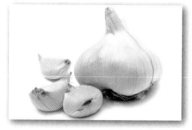

A WHITE WARRIOR. They're not just for slaying vampires—these mighty cloves are fantastic at fighting cancer and cardiovascular disease. While garlic may be rich in manganese, vitamin B6, vitamin C, and selenium, this member of the lily or *Allium* family has sulfur-containing compounds. One such compound, allicin, has been shown in studies to increase immunity and reduce colds by two-thirds. Early research also suggests that garlic consumption may actually help to regulate the number of fat cells that form in the body. Don't let the smell keep you away. Take a big bite today, and you may scare off a cold—and obesity.

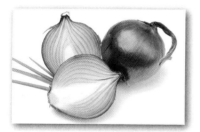

THE BONE BUILDER. Onions are loaded with numerous bone-building compounds. First, they contain something called F-L-glutamyl-trans-S-1-propenyl-L-cysteine sulfoxide that may inhibit the activity of cells responsible for breaking down bones. Onions also contain quercetin and kaempferol, two phytochemicals that may increase bone density. These white bone builders also promote bone health because they contain inulin, a plant fiber that has been shown to increase calcium absorption by 33 percent. So serving onions in a cream sauce may be a prescription for an osteoporosis-free future. These numerous nutrients may help to explain why the women of Turkey, who have the highest consumption of onions in the world, also have the lowest osteoporosis-related bone fracture rate in Europe.

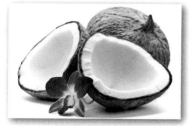

WEIGHT-LOSS WONDER. Not only does the liquid from a coconut contain all five of the same electrolytes as human blood (calcium, magnesium, potassium, sodium, and phosphorous), but the meat itself is quite a marvel. Coconuts contain a fantastic fat-fighting fat called MCT, or medium chain

PRODUCE

triglycerides. These healthy fats increase the oxidation of fat, allowing you to burn up body fat and lose fat fast! So, if you are working on your beach body, you might want to consider eating this tropical treat!

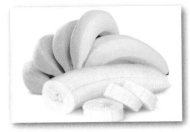

A BUNCH OF POTASSIUM. They may be yellow on the outside, but these white-fleshed fruits are packed with powerful potassium. Bananas are one of our best sources of powerful potassium, delivering over 450 mg in a single banana. Potassium is essential for maintaining normal blood pressure and heart function. Potassium is also critical for strong, healthy bones, as it helps to control pH levels in body fluids. Cranky from getting awakened by leg cramps? This potassium packer should be your pack-and-peel pick!

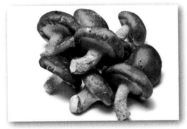

EXCEPTIONAL ANTIOXIDANTS. There is fungus among us, and it is jam-packed with heart-healthy properties. In fact, crimini mushrooms—the most common and familiar variety—have been shown in recent studies to have more antioxidant benefits than some of the exotic mushroom counterparts. These caps provide an excellent source of selenium, zinc, and manganese—all critical antioxidant nutrients—and are required for the functioning of antioxidant enzymes. Additionally, crimini mushrooms contain some unusual antioxidant molecules called ergothioneine, exceptional antioxidants that specifically help to prevent oxidative damage to DNA. And because your heart health depends on great antioxidant protection, it is not surprising to see crimini mushrooms providing impressive cardiovascular benefits. So caps off to the antioxidant-rich fungi!

Proper Produce Preparation

NOW THAT YOU'VE MADE THE DECISION to add a brilliant color palette of local, organic produce to your daily diet, we want to ensure you lock in all the nutritional benefits possible. To do so, let's review proper produce preparation. Is it best to eat foods raw or cooked? Should we peel our vegetables or eat them with skins on? Here are a few guidelines that will help you to make the best decisions you can about how to prepare your precious produce.

Raw or Cooked?

TOMATOES: We mentioned earlier that tomatoes are an excellent source of the cancer fighter lycopene. They are also a fantastic source of vitamin C, an antioxidant that fights cell-damaging free radicals, and folate, a promoter of healthy red blood cells and anti-Alzheimer's aid. While both vitamin C and folate are preserved best without heat, cooked tomatoes contain three to four times more lycopene than raw ones. The lycopene gets locked in the fibrous portion of vegetables, and cooking releases it. What to do? Eat tomatoes in salads to capture the full spectrum of micronutrients, and enjoy them heated in Italian dishes to ensure maximum lycopene delivery.

GARLIC: We want to make sure that this healthful powerhouse delivers all of its anti-cancer, heart-protective, fat-cell–regulating, and immunity-boosting properties. The bad news is that its health-promoting compounds are destroyed when heated, and garlic can be a bit pungent when eaten raw. The good news is that there is a two-step plan to help you lock in these vital sulfur compounds. First, chop or crush the garlic at least ten minutes before adding it to heat to stimulate the enzymatic process that converts the phytonutrient alliin to allicin, the compound to which many of garlic's health benefits are attributed. Next, add the garlic to a recipe fifteen minutes before it is ready to be served to reduce long-term heat exposure.

CRUCIFEROUS VEGETABLES: Cruciferous (meaning "cross bearing") vegetables have flowers that resemble the shape of a cross: arugula, bok choy, broccoli, brussels sprouts, cabbage, cauliflower, collard greens, kale, radish, rutabaga, turnip, and watercress. This family of vegetables contains compounds that can compete with iodine for uptake by the thyroid gland. So, if you are concerned about slugging thyroid function, you should cook your cruciferous vegetables to reduce these goitrogenic substances by about two-thirds.

GREENS: Enjoy the outstanding micronutrient benefits of leafy greens, but make sure the majority of your consumption is cooked. As mentioned in the Everyday Micronutrient Depleter section, spinach, chard, parsley, chives, and beet greens all contain an anti-nutrient called oxalic acid. Oxalic acid binds to calcium, magnesium, and iron, robbing you of the micronutrients you expect your food to deliver. Additionally, consuming these foods raw on a regular basis may cause the eventual formation of kidney stones. Research has shown that by boiling spinach in large amounts of water helps decrease the oxalic acid content by as much as 50 percent.

MUSHROOMS: Do you remember earlier when we told you about antioxidant compounds in the cells of crimini mushrooms called ergothioneine that help preserve DNA? Well, cooking your mushrooms rather than eating them raw actually releases this powerful nutrient from the mushroom cells, providing you with the promised protection. But that isn't the only reason to cook the caps. Agaritine, a potential carcinogen most concentrated in the mushroom caps, decompresses readily upon cooking (up to 90 percent reduction). That makes two great reasons to fire up the fungus.

Skin On or Skin Off?

While the fruits and vegetables you consume are just loaded with micronutrients and other health-promoting compounds, you may be surprised to know that those varieties with edible skins have tremendous micronutrient content in the skin. This is why we often tell people to put away their peelers. However, if the produce in question is one of the Fab Fourteen, and you opted to save some dough and buy it conventionally, you may be better off using that peeler after all. While the produce may have had limited exposure to pesticides, why take any chances? The rule of thumb here is that if the produce is organic, leave the peel on. If not, peel off. Either way, you want to make sure you wash it well before storing it in your fridge or fruit bowl.

Even fruit like citrus and melons needs to be washed well, even though you peel off or cut through the skin or rind. Why? Let's imagine you are going to cut a honeydew melon. First, consider how many hands have touched it, how many bugs have crawled over it, and how much dust has settled on it along its long journey to your home. Next, imagine the clean knife from your kitchen running through that microscopically filthy rind, cutting through the meat of the melon that you are about to serve to your family and friends. Now, pull the knife back through the same cut, further spreading bacteria. Next, make another cut. You get it now? It is important to thoroughly wash all fruits and vegetables, regardless of type.

A study by *Cook's Illustrated* examined four different cleaning techniques for produce: 1. A diluted vinegar solution followed by rinsing with cold water, 2. Antibacterial soap, 3. A water scrub with a brush, and 4. Rinsed with

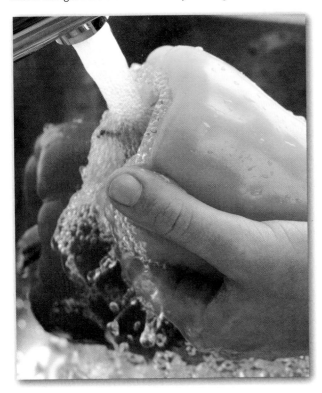

water. The results showed that the scrub brush with water removed 85 percent of unwanted bacteria (a little more than water alone), but the vinegar rinse removed 98 percent of bacteria on the surface of fresh fruits and vegetables. Interestingly, the study recommended against the use of antibacterial soap because of the ingredient triclosan. This agent, found in many antibacterial soaps, is believed to have the potential to eventually breed drug-resistant bacteria. If you want the most benefit from washing, it looks like water alone isn't the trick.

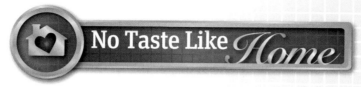

Vegetable Spray Wash

Don't waste your money on expensive vegetable washes. Make one yourself, and spray away the unwanted pesticides, wax coating, and bacteria.

INGREDIENTS

- 1 cup water
- 1 cup organic white vinegar
- 1 Tbsp. baking soda
- Juice of half a lemon

DIRECTIONS

 Mix ingredients in a tall pitcher to allow space for baking soda's "foam eruption" that occurs after vinegar is added.

 Spray on fruit, wait ten minutes, and wash off with cool water.

 Store in an empty spray bottle.

 Enjoy your clean, safe, delicious produce.

Frozen and Canned Produce

BELIEVE IT OR NOT, frozen or canned fruits and vegetables often start out with higher levels of micronutrients than their fresh counterparts because they are more likely to be picked at their peak of ripeness, when they are at their most micronutrient dense. Remember, fresh produce is often picked prior to peak ripeness to allow it to ripen during transport without becoming damaged or spoiled before arriving to the supermarket. However, it doesn't take long before this advantage is lost. During the blanching process—the soaking of the vegetables in hot water, which takes place prior to the freezing process—the micronutrient content of many of the water-soluble vitamins is reduced by an average of 20 to 60 percent. Loss of antioxidants (which are needed to fight free radicals) also occurs in the blanching and freezing process of most vegetables. While some of the micronutrients are lost, the good news is that the rest are locked into the frozen vegetables for up to twelve months.

Similarly, in canned foods, heat- and light-sensitive micronutrients can be lost through the cooking process prior to canning. However, once the can is sealed, the micronutrients that remain are stable for approximately two years. Researchers at the University of California, Davis, put it this way: "While the initial thermal treatment of canned products can result in loss, nutrients are relatively stable during subsequent storage due to the lack of oxygen. Frozen products lose fewer nutrients initially because of the short heating time in blanching, but they lose more nutrients during storage due to oxidation."

The losses incurred due to canning and freezing are similar to the data on micronutrient loss in vegetables during the first few weeks after being picked, when they would most likely be transported to the grocery store produce section. According to the UK-based Institute of Food Research, after just fifteen days, freshly picked green beans lost 45 percent of their total micronutrients, broccoli and cauliflower 25 percent, peas up to 15 percent, and carrots 10 percent.

So from a micronutrient standpoint, here is the rule of thumb: if your produce comes from local farmers and you it eat right away, you're better off buying it fresh. However, if you see in the supermarket produce section that the "fresh" vegetables come from some place far away, then there is a good chance that the vegetables in your grocer's frozen or canned vegetable aisles may be just as micronutrient dense.

We must now consider the safety of this prepackaged produce. Because the pesticide and GMO risk is the same regardless of fresh, canned, or frozen, the same rules apply when determining which to buy—organic or conventional. But unlike the fresh produce, these packaged counterparts often add some unwanted hazards in the forms of Poor Food ingredients and EMDs. Make sure when choosing frozen and canned foods to investigate the ingredients closely.

Many packaged foods contain high levels of sugar (EMD) and refined sodium, and most canned foods still comes in potentially dangerous BPA-lined cans. Keep in mind that tomatoes tend to leach BPA due to their high acidity, so make sure to always buy canned tomatoes in a BPA-free can or in a BPA-free self-stable container. Glass jars are great alternatives to cans, but make sure they are amber or opaque to protect your food from the store lights, which deplete its precious micronutrients. . . . And don't forget to recycle.

● ● ● ● ● ● ● ● ● ● ● ● ● ● ●

Fermented Produce

WHEN WE THINK OF FERMENTATION, we often think of wine or beer, but food can be fermented, too. In fact, it is another great way to prepare and preserve your produce. Fermentation is the act of using bacteria, molds, and/or yeasts to create alcohol, acetic acid, or lactic acid, which then act as natural preservatives for food and its micronutrients. Fermentation can add exciting, complex flavors to food and can even create new vitamins, especially B-vitamins and K2, but sadly, it can also deplete others. The big benefit to fermented foods is that over time, they can improve the health and efficiency of your gut. In other words, they can create an environment where proper digestion and nutrient absorption can take place. They accomplish this by stimulating the gut to produce hydrochloric acid, which is essential for both processes and can eliminate acid reflux naturally. Eating fermented produce such as kimchi, sauerkraut, cortido, or just about anything pickled can reduce or eliminate the need for digestive aids, and work to increase the population of healthy flora throughout your intestine, which reduces the need for pricey probiotics.

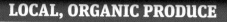

STEER HERE

LOCAL, ORGANIC PRODUCE

- Fresh/local
- Organic

FROZEN

CASCADIAN FARMS BOXED, BAGGED AND PREMIUM BLENDS FROZEN VEGETABLES (EXCEPT FRENCH-CUT GREEN BEANS WITH TOASTED ALMONDS, AND PURELY STEAM BROCCOLI & CARROTS AND GARDEN VEGETABLE MEDLEY)

- Organic
- Frozen at peak ripeness

SAFEWAY O ORGANICS FROZEN VEGETABLES (ALL VARIETIES)

- Organic
- Frozen at peak ripeness

PACKAGED FRUIT

NATIVE FOREST TROPICAL FRUIT SALAD

- Organic
- BPA free
- Sugar free

SANTA CRUZ ORGANIC APPLESAUCE (NO SUGAR ADDED)

- Organic
- BPA-free glass jar
- Sugar free

PUBLIX GREENWISE MARKET ORGANIC UNSWEETENED APPLE SAUCE

- Organic
- BPA free
- Sugar free

CANNED VEGETABLES

NATIVE FOREST ORGANIC (ALL VARIETIES EXCEPT CANNED MUSHROOMS)

- Organic
- BPA-free
- Canned at peak ripeness

PRODUCE

TOMATO PRODUCTS

EDEN ORGANIC TOMATOES IN AMBER GLASS (ALL VARIETIES)

- Organic
- BPA safe
- Amber glass protected

NATURAL VALUE TOMATOES (ALL VARIETIES)

- Organic
- BPA-free cans for all tomato products

MUIR GLEN ORGANIC CANNED TOMATO PASTE

- Organic
- Nothing but tomato
- BPA-free cans now in production (if the can's interior does not have a white lining, it is a new BPA-free can)

FERMENTED PRODUCE

BUBBIES PURE KOSHER DILLS

- Sugar free
- No added vinegar

Also try their delicious and mild sauerkraut.

REJUVENATIVE SPICY KIM-CHI

- Organic
- No sugar added

Try all of their fantastic raw, organic cultured vegetables.

EDEN ORGANIC SAUERKRAUT

- Organic
- No added sugar

FROZEN

GREEN GIANT BROCCOLI & CHEESE SAUCE

The front of the package looks so promising, with the "Picked at the Peak of Perfection" across the top, a Weight Watchers endorsement badge, and boldly in blue the words "60 calories per serving." But turn it over, and the nightmare begins. Not only are there two and a half servings in the small 10-ounce box, there are also over twenty-five ingredients in this seemingly simple broccoli and cheese, and that is not counting the twelve ingredients that make up the three kinds of cheeses! Dieters and families alike will want to beware of this product's modified cornstarch (GMO), BHA (probable carcinogen), partially hydrogenated soybean oil (GMO, trans fat), corn syrup solids (EMD, GMO), whey protein concentrate (MSG), hydrolyzed corn gluten (MSG, GMO), artificial flavors, autolyzed yeast extract (MSG), dextrose (GMO sugar), and added color (we are assuming it is not natural). Both Green Giant and Weight Watchers should know better.

PACKAGED FRUIT

MOTT'S STRAWBERRY APPLESAUCE

Start with a non-organic variety of the fruit highest on the Terrible Twenty and add in high fructose corn syrup (GMO/EMD) and red #40. If the sugar isn't enough to overexcite your children, the counterfeit color should do the trick.

DEL MONTE 100-CALORIE FRUIT COCKTAIL

They may offer you portion control, but someone needs to teach Del Monte ingredient control. This non-organic fruit cup coats five fruits with three forms of sweeteners: acesulfame potassium and sucralose (both SSS) and sugar (EMD). Top it off with artificially colored cherries and package it in a BPA-lined can, and this diet treat sounds more like a disaster.

CANNED VEGETABLES

GLORY FOODS SENSIBLY SEASONED MIXED GREENS

These "sensible" greens may be certified by the American Heart Association, but they must not have looked at the ingredient list. These water-logged, non-organic greens contain hydrolyzed soy protein (MSG, GMO), caramel color (possible carcinogen), and sugar (EMD)—not to mention the fact that they are sitting in a BPA-lined can.

TOMATO PRODUCTS

CONTADINA ITALIAN TOMATO PASTE WITH HERBS

Just like mama made, right? Not unless your mama worked in a high fructose corn syrup factory—and that's only the start of the nonsense. We have no idea why there are more than fifteen ingredients in this BPA-lined can, including GMO partially hydrogenated oils (trans fats), soy flour (GMO), and soy and wheat gluten. You will find better tomato paste options in Aisle 6, under pasta and pasta sauces.

FERMENTED FOODS

CLAUSSEN KOSHER DILL SANDWICH SLICES

You'll end up in a pickle if you choose these dills. The cucumbers are pickled in non-organic vinegar (think GMO corn), then tossed with high fructose corn syrup (GMO sugar), irradiated spices, and sodium benzoate (possible carcinogen).

☐ Choose local, organic if available.

☐ Choose organic whenever budget allows.

☐ Choose organic if buying any of the Terrible Twenty.

☐ Choosing frozen or canned produce is an option when produce is not in season or was grown far from your home.

☐ Choose BPA-free packaging.

☐ Avoid added ingredients, including sugar, coloring, and refined sodium.

☐ Avoid bacteria, pesticide residue, and wax by washing all produce, whether preparing with or without skin.

My go-to Rich Food choices for produce: _____

_____

_____

_____

_____

_____

_____

_____

_____

_____

_____

_____

_____

PRODUCE

Aisle FIVE

Condiments

S mack dab in the middle of the market await numerous flavorings to top the foods we have already purchased. It's too bad that all of our due diligence shopping the store's perimeter, thus far to stock up on the most micronutrient-rich foods, can be sabotaged simply with a few condiment criminals lurking in this aisle. Adding a dab or a dollop of an inferior product will bring the good stuff down with it. What is really unfortunate is these condiments were once innocent—that is, before manufacturers destroyed them. As we push our cart down the condiments aisle, from mayonnaise and salad dressings to peanut butters and jellies, there are few options that meet our Rich Food criteria. But we've still managed to wean out a few of the better options and offer homemade fresh recipes that meet our standards.

Mayonnaise, Tartar Sauce, and Horseradish

THE FRENCH CREATED MAYONNAISE in the 1700s as a simple emulsion of eggs, oil, and either lemon juice or vinegar, so why do we find thickening agents, gels, GMO oils, and sweeteners jammed into the jars sold to us today?

In a perfect world, mayonnaise would be made with either olive oil or coconut oil, or possibly a combination of the two. Most mayonnaises on the market today, however, use canola or soybean oil—two major GMO-laden pro-inflammatory no-nos! Even mayonnaise with "olive oil" proudly adorning the label, like Spectrum Organic Olive Oil or Hellman's Olive Oil, contains primarily either canola or soybean oil. Manufacturers try to fool us, but a simple inspection of the ingredients reveals that there is more Poor Food canola/soybean oil than the touted Rich Food olive oil—a case of a *made with* misleading misfit.

Organic canola and soybean oil are no better. While they are GMO free, these oils are highly processed man-made oils that contribute to the pro-inflammatory omega-6: omega-3 imbalance in our modern diets. (For more on choosing the best oil, see Aisle 7: Baking.) Additionally, it is nearly impossible to find a single mayonnaise that doesn't contain sugar.

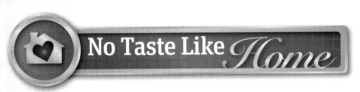

Five-Minute Mayonnaise

You'll never buy bottled or jarred again after tasting this marvelous Five-Minute Mayonnaise. By using the healthiest ingredients, you'll be the talk of the town with the best spread around.

INGREDIENTS

- 2 large pastured egg yolks
- 1 large pastured whole egg
- ½ tsp. organic mustard powder
- ¼ tsp. organic pepper (traditionally white pepper)
- ¼ tsp. unrefined sea salt

- 1 Tbsp. lemon juice *or* organic apple cider vinegar
- ½ cup organic cold-pressed extra virgin olive oil
- ½ cup organic extra virgin coconut oil (melted but not hot)

DIRECTIONS

 Making mayonnaise is an exercise in patience. While the recipe only takes five minutes, you can't rush the whisking process or the whole batch will be a waste. You can choose to whisk by hand, but unless your wrists are ready for a workout, it's best to opt for either a blender or a handheld immersion blender. We use a traditional blender, and it is perfect every time with no effort at all.

 Remove eggs from refrigerator and bring them to room temperate. Never attempt to make mayonnaise using chilled eggs.

 Combine eggs, mustard, salt, pepper, and your choice of either lemon juice or apple cider vinegar until smooth. Use a high blender speed for only fifteen seconds. Don't over mix.

 Combine the organic cold pressed extra virgin olive oil and organic extra virgin coconut oils in an easy-to-pour measuring cup.

 Slowly add approximately one half tablespoon of the oil into the egg mixture through the hole in the top of the blender while blending at low speed. Then add the other half. *We can't emphasize enough how slowly to add the oil.* Repeat this three more times. Your mixture should be thickening now.

 Now your mixture should be ready to pour the oil in *slowly*. Create a thin stream of oil that is slowly incorporated into the blending egg mixture. You can now increase the blender's speed to medium high.

Once all of the oil has been mixed in, you will have a creamy, smooth homemade mayonnaise. If you add in the oil too quickly, you will have an oily spread that cannot be saved. Patience is a virtue, but your taste buds will be deliciously rewarded.

(By the way, this mayonnaise makes a fantastic moisturizer for damaged hair.)

Still think this sounds difficult? Come to the Rich Food Resource Center and watch the video that takes you step by step through this mayo-making process.

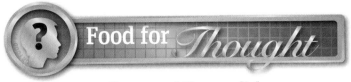

Food for *Thought*

Tartar and Horseradish

These tangier toppings fall fate to many of the same Poor Food ingredients. While they add flavor to your meal, don't allow them to be your downfall. Plan ahead and bottle your own. Horseradish is simply grated horseradish root with mayonnaise, and tartar takes that same homemade mayonnaise base and mixes in pickles, onion, and lemon juice. Looking for a low-fat alternative? Try mixing in zero-fat Greek yogurt in lieu of mayonnaise. Who would have thought all these condiments could be created in your kitchen?!

STEER HERE

OUR TOP PICKS! Homemade Five-Minute Mayonnaise and Homemade Tartar and Horseradish

MAYONNAISE

WILDERNESS FAMILY NATURALS ORGANIC MAYONNAISE

- Organic olive, coconut, and sesame seed oil
- Still contains minimal evaporated cane juice (sugar)

HOT HORSERADISH

TRUE NATURAL TASTE HOT HORSERADISH

- Organic horseradish
- Organic apple cider vinegar

STEER CLEAR

HELLMAN'S LIGHT MAYONNAISE

You may be trying to reduce the calories, but by picking this spread, you just increased your intake of Poor Food ingredients. The soybean oil base (GMO) adds in high fructose corn syrup (EMD, GMO), phosphoric acid (EMD), and modified corn-starch (GMO). On top of that, the first ingredient listed is water—simply an ingredient you shouldn't be wasting your money on. Kraft and Hellman's regular mayonnaises aren't much better—they still contain soybean oil (GMO) and sugar (EMD).

KRAFT TARTAR SAUCE FAT FREE

Don't ruin your wild-caught fish with this Poor Food condiment. It is made of non-organic white vinegar (GMO), sugar (EMD), modified food starch (GMO), high fructose corn syrup (EMD), soybean oil (GMO), cellulose gel, artificial flavor, coloring chameleons (yellow #6, blue #1), and calcium disodium EDTA (EMD). Make your own!

BEAVER CREAM STYLE HORSERADISH SAUCE

This company is horsing around! Their horseradish sauce contains white distilled vinegar (GMO), high fructose corn syrup (EMD, GMO), fructose (sugar), sugar (EMD), soybean oil (GMO), disodium EDTA (EMD), and sodium benzoate (possible carcinogen).

❑ Choose to make your own mayonnaise, tartar, and horseradish with Rich Food ingredients.

❑ Choose organic.

❑ Choose olive oil and/or coconut oil.

❑ Avoid sugars.

❑ Avoid canola, soybean, and sunflower oil.

My go-to Rich Food choices for mayonnaise, tartar sauce, and horseradish sauce: _____

_____

_____

_____

_____

_____

_____

_____

_____

Checkout Checklist

Ketchup and Mustard

THESE TOPPINGS just make your burger better. Add our Five-Minute Mayonnaise, and your bun will burst with flavor. (For more information on rolls and buns, see Aisle 6: Grains.) But beware—grocery store ketchup is filled with added sugar. And since tomatoes aren't on the Fabulous Fourteen, we should make every effort to find organic varieties of this tomato topper. Organic ketchup is a Rich Food powerhouse because it has three times the amount of cancer-preventing lycopene as conventional ketchup.

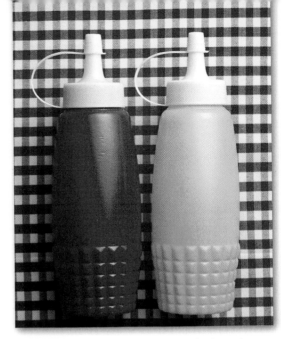

For mustard, the rule is the same—buy organic. Mustard is a mixture of distilled white vinegar and spices. White vinegar in conventional mustard is usually derived from corn, so you become susceptible to GMOs. Additionally, the spices will have been irradiated in the brand-name mustards, and we want to steer clear of these free radical–causing Everyday Micronutrient Depleters.

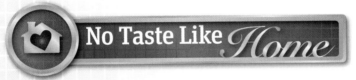

No Taste Like Home

Killer Ketchup That Won't Kill You

This is a *ketchup* recipe that has *caught up* to the times.
It is sugar free, organic, and stores well in the refrigerator.

INGREDIENTS

- 12 oz. can of organic tomato paste (remember to look for BPA-free cans)
- ½ cup water
- 2 Tbsp. organic white vinegar
- ½ tsp. organic garlic powder

- 1 tsp. organic onion powder
- 1 tsp. organic all spice
- Organic cayenne pepper to taste
- Unrefined sea salt and organic pepper to taste

- Pure stevia extract (or preferred sugar substitute) to taste (for more about Rich Food sweeteners, see Aisle 7)

DIRECTIONS

1 Combine ingredients in a saucepan over medium heat, and stir until smooth.

2 Cool and store in canning jar (preferably opaque) and refrigerate.

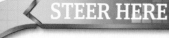

STEER HERE

OUR TOP PICK! Homemade Killer Ketchup

KETCHUP

REJUVENATIVE RAW LIVE KETCHUP

● Organic ● High lycopene content ● Sugar free ● Probiotic

They also make a sweeter version flavored with honey for those so inclined.

MUIR GLEN ORGANIC KETCHUP

● Organic ● High lycopene content ● Still contains sugar

WEGMANS ORGANIC KETCHUP

● Organic ● High lycopene content ● Still contains sugar

ANNIE'S ORGANIC KETCHUP

● Organic ● High lycopene content ● Still contains sugar

MUSTARD

ANNIE'S ORGANIC YELLOW MUSTARD

● Organic ● Sugar free

EDEN BROWN MUSTARD

● Organic ● Sugar free

KETCHUP

HEINZ

America's favorite ketchup is a bottle bomb. Their non-organic tomatoes are not only likely coated with pesticides but also with corn-derived distilled vinegar (GMO), high fructose corn syrup (EMD, GMO), corn syrup (GMO), irradiated spices (EMD), and natural flavorings (most likely MSG). Dressing your quality grass-fed beef burger with this Poor Food tomato topper would be a sin. Heinz Organic still contains sugar and natural flavorings (MSG), so choose one of our Steer Here selected brands.

MUSTARD

GREY POUPON DIJON MUSTARD

Don't be fooled into thinking this fancier mustard is a smarter choice. It is made with non-organic vinegar (GMO), irradiated spices (EMD), and added sugar (EMD). As *our* saying goes, "Pass *on* the Grey Poupon!"

Checkout Checklist

❑ Choose to make your own Killer Ketchup.
❑ Choose organic.
❑ Avoid sugars.
❑ Avoid irradiated spices.
❑ Avoid non-organic vinegar.

My go-to Rich Food choices for ketchup and mustard: _____

_____

_____

_____

_____

Salsa and Guacamole

WHILE THESE PRODUCTS OFTEN APPEAR on the plate together, accompanying your fiery fajitas or atop your tasty taco salad, one of them is easily found in the supermarket as a Rich Food, while the other is best made at home. Salsa is the number one selling condiment in the United States, and whether you prefer it mild or spicy, it follows the same rule as ketchup, because its base is also tomato. But it is even more important to purchase organic salsa because sweet peppers and hot peppers, two common salsa ingredients, are on the Terrible Twenty. Luckily, there are a lot of Rich Food organic salsa options in the supermarkets today. Guacamole, on the other hand, is more problematic. Many offerings are loaded with fake ingredients, and some are even canned and stacked on the shelf next to the chips. Stick with fresh varieties in the refrigerated section, and examine the label to be sure there are no Poor Food ingredients—or try the following Holy Moly recipe at home.

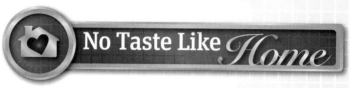

Holy Moly Guacamole!

You'll be ready to start the fiesta when you finish making this quick and easy recipe, but don't dig in too *rapido*. The guacamole flavors need time to meld. Allow it to sit in the refrigerator for thirty minutes before dipping in—if you can!

INGREDIENTS

- 2 ripe avocados
- 1 small onion
- 1 garlic clove
- 1 ripe organic tomato
- 1 lime, juiced
- Organic jalapeno peppers, minced for seasoning to taste
- Unrefined sea salt and organic pepper to taste

DIRECTIONS

 1 Peel the avocados and remove the pits.

 2 Peel and mince the onion and garlic.

 3 Chop the tomato and the optional jalapeno.

 4 Mash the avocado in the bowl and stir in the onion, garlic, tomato, and jalapeno.

 5 Season with the lime juice and salt and pepper.

 6 Chill for thirty minutes before serving.

OPTION:
In a hurry? Take the mashed avocado and simply add 2 tablespoons of organic salsa instead of all of the other ingredients. It isn't quite homemade, but its starts the fiesta real fast!

STEER HERE

Coupon Clipper

SALSA

REJUVENATIVE LIVE GREEN SALSA

- Organic
- Active cultures
- Celtic salt
- Tomato free

MUIR GLEN MEDIUM SALSA

- Organic
- Sugar free
- Multiple flavors available

AMY'S FIRE ROASTED VEGETABLE SALSA

- Organic
- Sugar free
- Multiple flavors available

GUACAMOLE

OUR TOP PICK! Homemade Holy Moly Guacamole

Coupon Clipper

WHOLLY ORGANIC GUACAMOLE

- Organic
- Sugar free

STEER CLEAR

SALSA

OLD EL PASO ALL NATURAL THICK N' CHUNKY MILD SALSA

Take a pass on the old El Paso. Non-organic tomatoes (low lycopene) with non-organic vinegar (GMO), jalapenos (pesticides), irradiated spices (EMD), and, of course . . . sugar.

TEXAS ON THE PLATE, CAMPFIRE CORN SALSA

When non-organic corn is in the name, GMOs are on your plate. Add to the jar two types of peppers (possible pesticide *problemas!*), lime zest in the form of lime and added sugar (according to the ingredient list), and it's lights out for this campfire salsa.

GUACAMOLE

LAURA SCUDDER'S GUACAMOLE DIP

It takes forty-four ingredients to make this green toxic mush. There isn't even any whole avocado in the recipe. Laura uses GMO canola oil, MSG-laden modified food starch, non-organic peppers, and trans fat containing GMO partially hydrogenated soybean oil—plus irradiated, free-radical loaded spices, GMO corn syrup solids, possibly carcinogenic caramel color, GMO soy sauce, micronutrient-depleting sugar, obesity-inducing monosodium glutamate, and the counterfeit colors yellow #5 and blue #1.

☐ **Choose organic salsa.**

☐ **Choose to make make homemade Holy Moly Guacamole.**

☐ Avoid added sugars and artificial colors.

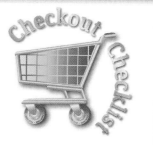

My go-to Rich Food choices for salsa and guacamole: _____

_____

_____

_____

Salad Dressing

HERE AGAIN, WE ALMOST STRUCK OUT. Conventional grocery stores didn't have any-thing—not *one* product—that satisfied *all* of our Rich Food requirements, even when they were organic. As with mayonnaise, most salad dressings use cheap GMO sources of oils such as canola and soybean oil that we want to avoid. Manufacturers obviously assume we want our vegetables coated in sugar because the dressing on the store shelves adds in sugar, high fructose corn syrup, corn syrup solids, maltodex-trin, and fruit juice concentrates.

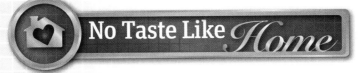

Don't settle for drab dressings with inferior ingredients.
Tantalize your taste buds with these do-it-yourself dressings.

Really Creamy Blue Cheese Dressing (or Dip)

INGREDIENTS

- ¾ cup organic raw blue cheese, crumbled
- 3 oz. organic cream cheese, softened
- ½ cup mayonnaise (use our Five-Minute Mayonnaise, page 152)
- ⅓ cup organic sour cream

DIRECTIONS

1. Combine with immersion blender and store in a sealed glass canning jar (opaque).

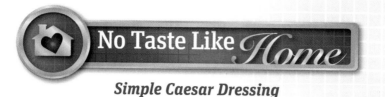

Simple Caesar Dressing

INGREDIENTS

- 1 Tbsp. lemon juice
- ½ tsp. organic ground pepper
- ½ tsp. unrefined sea salt
- ½ tsp. organic garlic powder or 2 cloves garlic, minced
- ¼ cup organic cold pressed extra-virgin olive oil

- ½ cup freshly grated organic Parmesan cheese (for a guide to purchasing cheese, see page 75)
- 1 large pastured egg yolk
- 5 anchovies, chopped (or 1 tsp. anchovies paste. Both a great added source of omega-3)
- Organic red wine vinegar to taste

DIRECTIONS

 1 Combine and blend ingredients (with the exception of the red wine vinegar) using a handheld immersion blender.

 2 Use a piece of lettuce to taste the dressing.

3 Adjust acid level by adding red wine vinegar to the dressing.

4 Pour over romaine lettuce and top with Parmesan cheese shavings.

Zesty Avocado Dressing (or Dip)

INGREDIENTS

- 1 ripe avocado (peeled and cored)
- 1 cup plain organic Greek yogurt (fat free or full fat for a creamier dressing)
- 2 green onions, finely chopped
- 3 Tbsp. lime juice (about 1.5 limes, juiced)
- 1 tsp. lime zest (or zest of one lime)
- 2 Tbsp. organic cold-pressed extra virgin olive oil

- 1 garlic clove, minced
- ½ tsp. organic cumin
- ½ tsp. unrefined sea salt
- ½ tsp. organic pepper
- Organic cayenne pepper to taste (we use ½ tsp.)

DIRECTIONS

 1 Combine with immersion blender, and store in a sealed glass canning jar (opaque).

Fantastic as a dip for baked veggie chips on page 231!

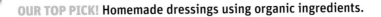

STEER HERE

OUR TOP PICK! Homemade dressings using organic ingredients.

SALAD DRESSING

VIGOA CUISINE LIME SPLASH

- Organic • Made with cold pressed extra-virgin olive oil
- Celtic sea salt • Makes a fantastic marinade and dip

Also available in Garlic and Herb Splash and Hot Splash

ZUKAY SWEET ONION BASIL DRESSING

- Oil free dressing • Live active cultures • Celtic sea salt
- Some organic ingredients • Makes a fantastic marinade and dip

Also available in five other unique probiotic flavors.

TESSEMAE'S ALL NATURAL DRESSINGS

- Extra virgin olive oil • Some organic ingredients
- Organic (non-irradiated) spices

The most popular dressing is their classic, the Lemon Garlic.

STEER CLEAR

KRAFT CATALINA DRESSING

Four tablespoons of this dressing adds in almost as much sugar as an Almond Joy candy bar. The first ingredient is high fructose corn syrup (GMO), and the rest of the recipe includes soybean oil (GMO), phosphoric acid (EMD), disodium EDTA (EMD), and guar gum (EMD). You'll be flabbergasted when you realize that the vivid color comes compliments of heaping doses of counterfeit colors (red #40, yellow #6, blue #1).

GIRARD'S CAESAR SALAD DRESSING

The fancy gourmet bottle hides a plethora of Poor Food ingredients. If you enjoy soybean oil (GMO), corn cider vinegar (GMO), non-organic cheese (likely rBGH), and sugar (EMD), then pour on this dressing. As an extra bonus, it adds in three MSG-like substances, caramel color (possible carcinogen), and EDTA (EMD). They certainly have ruined this traditional Roman offering.

☐ Choose to make your own salad dressings with Rich Food ingredients.

☐ Choose organic.

☐ Choose organic cold pressed extra-virgin olive oil or coconut oil.

☐ Avoid sugars.

☐ Avoid canola, soybean, and sunflower oil.

☐ Avoid MSG, added colors, thickeners, and preservatives.

*My go-to Rich Food choices for salad dressing:*_____

_____

_____

_____

_____

_____

_____

• • • • • • • • • • • • •

Peanut Butter and Jelly

JUST THE MENTION OF PEANUT BUTTER AND JELLY conjures up fond childhood memories. When it comes to these comfort food condiments, picking the right peanut butters and jellies is far from child's play.

Peanut Butter and Other Nut Butters

There are four things you need to keep in mind when choosing the best peanut butter.

1 Try for an organic spread because peanuts are naturally high in fat and oil, and that makes them sponges for unwanted chemicals such as pesticides.

2 Find a peanut butter, like those we suggest under Steer Here, made from sprouted nuts. Remember, peanuts are considered plant seeds, and when a plant seed undergoes germination through sprouting or soaking, a lot of beneficial changes occur. The phytic acid

(EMD) that they naturally contain is broken down, which makes them far less micronutrient depleting. Also, their protease inhibitors, meant to protect them from insects, are inactivated. This is great news because these same protease inhibitors can also prevent protease enzymes from digesting protein in the human digestive tract. This burdens the pancreas and is thought to perhaps cause pancreatic cancer. Finally, sprouted peanuts have increased availability of vitamins and minerals, which, after all, makes them our Rich Food choice.

3 Read the ingredients. There is no reason for added sugars, oil, or preservatives. Pure and simple is always best.

4 Go nutty! Try a variety of nut butters like almond butter, cashew butter, or decadent mixed nut butter. This is especially relevant if you or family members have a peanut allergy or are striving to follow a Primal/paleo dietary profile. Peanut allergies are quite common and many health-conscious eaters are wary of certain mild objections to peanut butter, such as a mold called aflatoxin that grows on peanuts (though it's greatly reduced in the processing into butter), and a moderate level of lectins (gut irritators) that can compromise digestive health. Furthermore, peanuts are technically legumes, not nuts, so Primal/paleo followers commonly pursue alternatives accordingly. Quality grocers offer a variety of delicious, healthful nut butters, including almond, cashew, tahini (sesame seed), and even macadamia nut butter. Macadamia nut butter, although hard to find and expensive, is the premier Rich Food choice since it contains mostly monounsaturated fats and won't compromise your omega-6: omega-3 balancing efforts like other nut butters. And don't forget the delicious coconut butter we introduced you to in the dairy aisle (see page 82). Coconut butter provides the health-boosting, hard-to-find medium chain triglycerides (MCT) that enhance fat metabolism and regulate appetite.

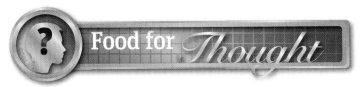

Food for Thought

Don't be fooled by the abundance of "natural" peanut butters on the market today. Remember in Chapter 3 we introduced you to this often misleading term used in marketing and packaging. While these nut spreads meet the government's guidelines for not containing synthetic ingredients, they do not assure you that they are safe or healthy. Many of these deceptive dips still load up on sugar, industrial oils, and other unpleasant EMDs.

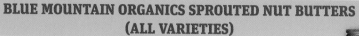

NUT BUTTERS

BLUE MOUNTAIN ORGANICS SPROUTED NUT BUTTERS (ALL VARIETIES)

- Organic
- Sprouted
- Contains one ingredient: nuts

We adore their sprouted macadamia nut butter!

WILDERNESS FAMILY NATURALS NUT BUTTERS (ALL VARIETIES)

- Organic
- Sprouted
- Contains one ingredient: nuts

ORGANIC NUTTZO

- Organic
- Mixed nuts with chia seeds and flax
- High omega-3

RAWMIO NUT BUTTER

- Organic
- Raw soaked hazelnuts
- Raw cocao nibs
- Raw coconut sugar
- Our go-to choice for a healthy Nutella alternative

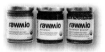

ARTISANA ORGANIC MACADAMIA-CASHEW BUTTER

- Organic
- Raw macadamias and cashews

SMUCKER'S ORGANIC PEANUT BUTTER

- Organic
- Contains one ingredient: nuts

STEER HERE

CONDIMENTS

NUT BUTTERS

JIF REDUCED FAT PEANUT BUTTER

Keep this one out of your cart. To make sure the unsprouted, non-organic peanuts are sweet enough, Jif peanuts are coated with corn syrup (GMO, EMD), sugar (EMD), and molasses (more sugar). Then, they add a soy protein (EMD, MSG) and mix it all up with soybean and canola oils (GMO) and mono and diglycerides (trans fat aliases). With seventeen ingredients, there's got to be a better butter!

NUTELLA

The name starts with the word *nut,* but the ingredients don't. Instead, sugar is the first ingredient. That means it isn't so much a nut spread as a sugar spread. Every serving, just two tablespoons, contains the same amount of sugar as two Reese's Peanut Butter Cups. That's nuts!

Jellies, Jams, Preserves, and Fruit Spreads

Adding sweetness to your morning, all these marvelous marmalades add unwanted Poor Food ingredients, too. Most of the fruits in these spreads (strawberries, blueberries, peaches, grapes) are on our Terrible Twenty (see page 132), which means they should always be purchased organic due to the probability of high pesticide residue.

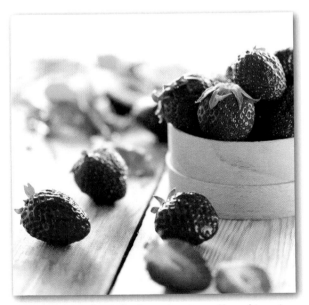

Additionally, we believe if you really want fruit, you should eat it whole. You can eat a dozen strawberries for the same amount of calories as one tablespoon of strawberry jelly or preserves. Eating real fruit avoids consuming added sugars or corn syrups and locks in more micronutrients—plus you'll feel much more satiated for longer periods of time while locking in much-needed fiber. Just think of how much more satisfying and filling a bowl of fresh strawberries would be—and you don't need a piece of bread to enjoy the fresh fruit option, either! (To find out why that's a good thing, hit Aisle 6: Grains.)

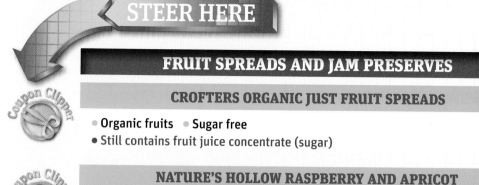

STEER HERE

FRUIT SPREADS AND JAM PRESERVES

CROFTERS ORGANIC JUST FRUIT SPREADS

- Organic fruits
- Sugar free
- Still contains fruit juice concentrate (sugar)

NATURE'S HOLLOW RASPBERRY AND APRICOT SUGAR-FREE JAM PRESERVES

- Sweetened with xylitol (sugar alcohol)
- While not organic, these fruits are not on the Terrible Twenty

STEER CLEAR

FRUIT SPREADS AND JAM PRESERVES

SMUCKER'S STRAWBERRY PRESERVES

With a name like Smucker's, it is supposed to be good, but one look at the label will quickly tell us otherwise. Strawberries top the Terrible Twenty, so this non-organic spread is not to be trusted. And it's loaded with high fructose corn syrup (GMO/EMD), sugar (EMD), and corn syrup (GMO). Smucker's should be smacked for putting 12 grams of sugar in every tablespoon—that's the equivalent of eight Everlasting Gobstoppers.

WELCH'S CONCORD GRAPE JELLY

No wonder this jelly is a favorite with most kids—you might as well have given them a candy bar! Each serving contains 13 grams of pure sugar (more than a fun-size 3 Musketeers bar) and of course is made with only the finest non-organic grapes (number 7 on the Terrible Twenty), corn syrup (GMO, EMD), and high fructose corn syrup (GMO, EMD). Time for a pantry purge!

POLANER REAL MINT JELLY

Don't ruin your organic grass-fed lamb chops with this minty madness! The first two ingredients are high fructose corn syrup (GMO, EMD) and corn syrup (GMO), followed by pectin (EMD), sugar (EMD), and two counterfeit colors (yellow #5 and blue#1). There isn't even any fruit to be found in this jelled spread.

Pancake Syrup

SUNDAY MORNING BRUNCH often comes with a plate of pancakes (see our wheat-free recipe on page 205), but short stacks beware—all syrups are not created equal. In this category, you will have to consider what kind of syrup you are buying as well as how much sugar you want in your diet. Steer clear of the typical name-brand syrups, and choose a 100 percent real maple syrup. However, if you are like us, and looking to lower your intake of sugar altogether, consider skipping it or saving it for rare occasions.

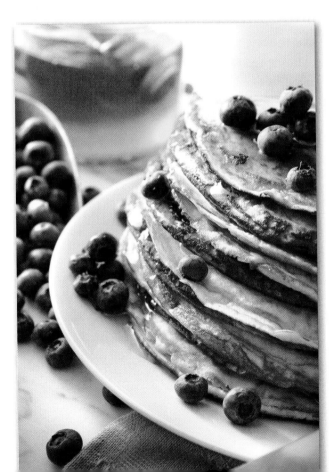

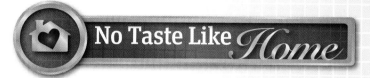

Move over maple—berry may just taste better! There is nothing better than fresh, local, organic berries straight from the farm. But this recipe can still be good using organic frozen ones. Served warm or cold, this antioxidant-rich syrup is sure to satisfy.

Triple Berry Syrup

INGREDIENTS

- 1 cup organic blueberries, fresh or frozen
- 1 cup organic raspberries
- 1 cup organic blackberries
- ½ cup water
- Pinch of unrefined sea salt

- Pure stevia extract (or preferred sugar substitute) to taste (For more about Rich Food sweeteners, see Aisle 7.)

DIRECTIONS

 1 Put ingredients in saucepan and bring to a boil. The berries will begin to soften and break apart as soon as the boiling begins.

 2 After five minutes, turn off heat. Use a potato masher or fork to mash or break down the remaining berries.

 3 Turn the heat back up and boil for another two minutes, while stirring to combine.

 4 Remove from heat. Your syrup will thicken as it cools.

5 Serve warm or refrigerate in canning jars.

This is also fantastic mixed with plain Greek yogurt, atop your favorite ice cream, or in lieu of jelly.

Watch the free video tutorial online in the Calton Nutrition Rich Food Resource Center. Pancakes and syrup have never been so simple . . . or healthy!

SYRUP

NATURE'S HOLLOW RASPBERRY SUGAR-FREE SYRUP

• Sugar free • Sweetened with xylitol (sugar alcohol) • Diabetic safe

MAPLE VALLEY ORGANIC MAPLE SYRUP U.S. GRADE B

For those occasions that call for 100 percent real maple syrup. • All natural

STEER CLEAR

SYRUP

AUNT JEMIMA ORIGINAL

This aunt is no *jem.* Your perfect pancakes deserve better that corn syrup (GMO, EMD), high fructose corn syrup (GMO, EMD), caramel color, sodium benzoate (two possible carcinogens), and artificial and natural flavors (MSG). This maple syrup imposter contains 32 grams of sugar in each serving—that's more than five rolls of Smarties candy.

MRS. BUTTERWORTH LITE

This syrup isn't worth *syrv*ing! Don't buy a lite syrup thinking you are getting better ingredients—what you're really paying for is the same Poor Food ingredients watered down with added thickeners. Water is the first ingredient in this mess, followed by sugar syrup (EMD), high fructose corn syrup (EMD, GMO), cellulose gum (to thicken), sodium benzoate and caramel color (two possible carcinogens), phosphoric acid (EMD), natural and artificial flavors (MSG), corn syrup (EMD, GMO), and molasses (sugar). It's lights out for this lite syrup.

☐ Choose to make homemade Triple Berry Syrup.

☐ Choose 100 percent maple syrup for special occasions if you aren't concerned about sugar content.

☐ Avoid syrups with long lists of Poor Food ingredients.

My go-to Rich Food choices for pancake syrup: _____

Aisle SIX

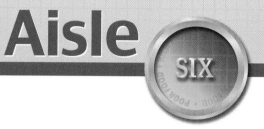

Grains

While there isn't a "grain" aisle in the supermarket, products made from grain have been the subject of much controversy and confusion, and therefore, we offer this compilation of grain foods in one demystifying section. Controversial because some of the biggest names in the food industry, like General Mills, Pepperidge Farm, Uncle Ben's, Barilla, and Quaker Oats, claim that whole grains—wheat, corn, rice, cereals, and others—used in their cereals, breads, rice dishes, and pastas are healthy. They are touted as a dietary centerpiece that boosts energy, fights cholesterol, and controls weight. On the other side of the debate, people like William Davis, MD, author of *Wheat Belly;* Mark Hyman, MD, author of the *Blood Sugar Solution;* and Mark Sisson, author of the *Primal Blueprint* and a leader in the evolutionary health movement, stress that grains, especially wheat, are destructive to good health.

So, whom should we listen to? Should we believe the huge food conglomerates that bring us foods like Lucky Charms and Chef Boyardee Beefaroni loaded with Poor Food ingredients? Or those who are on the front lines every day, working to find ways to improve the health of their patients and clients? We have seen tremendous improvements in our clients' health when they reduce or eliminate wheat and other grains from their diets. Unfortunately, becoming knowledgeable about the pitfalls of eating grains leaves little chance of finding traditional grain-based products that fit into your new dietary standards.

GRAINS

Grain Review

WHILE WE HAVE CHOSEN to eliminate most grains, including wheat, from our own diet and have advocated to more than ten thousand clients over twenty years to do the same, you may not be ready to entirely drain the grains from your diet just yet. And that's understandable, since for so many years, the USDA and low-fat proponents have been spreading propaganda about the benefits of "heart-healthy" low-fat, fiber-rich grain—recommending as much as eleven servings a day as the basis for a healthy diet.

If this anti-wheat commentary contradicts with your beliefs on grains that you have held near and dear for your entire life, you should reflect on the truth that the health advice the US government is promoting has been a widespread devastating failure. Residents of the United States and other Western nations following a grain-based diet are now the fattest population in the history of the Earth, and for the first time in recorded history, today's children have a lower life expectancy than their parents.

Since many of us are sick and tired of being sick and tired, and watching unlucky friends and loved ones suffer the consequences of eating the Standard American Diet (SAD), momentum is building in the direction of grain-free eating. Talk-show host and political pundit Bill O'Reilly has weaned the wheat and says, "My cholesterol has dropped big time. My indigestion, gone away. And so have my allergies." Thousands of individuals following low-carb and paleo diets have been living grain free. Numerous celebrities including *The View's* Elisabeth Hasselbeck, pop star Lady Gaga, fashion designer Rachel Roy, billionaire business tycoon Mark Cuban, actresses Jennifer Esposito and Rachel Weisz, and Super Bowl champion quarterback Drew Brees have all eliminated wheat from their diets and are boasting about their improved health.

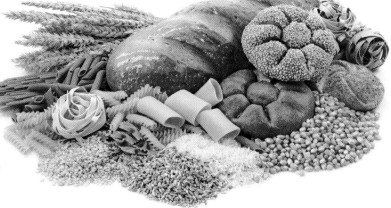

But before you can move any further to choosing, or not choosing, a box of cereal or a loaf of bread, we offer you our guide to grains to help you swiftly and smartly read ingredient lists and translate the misfit marketing that is plaguing the grain-heavy aisles.

Wheat

Foods made with wheat flour raise your blood sugar higher than almost any other food—more than sugar or even a candy bar! This goes for all forms of wheat across the board—organic, multigrain, sprouted—even the almighty "whole grains"—which is surprising to say the least. Let's learn why wheat is such a shock to our metabolic system. Ninety-nine percent of today's wheat is the result of an unhealthy, intense genetic manipulation of the wheat of our grandparents' generation. Stalks that were originally four feet tall—"amber waves of grain"—are now two-feet-tall dwarf stalks. This is thanks to over forty years of crude, imperfect gene manipulation by scientists that pre-dates what we consider today to be gene modification (GMO).

There are four main components that Wheat Belly author Dr. William Davis believes makes wheat so devastating to our health. The first is what's known as gliadin protein. Dr. Davis explains, "The gliadin protein is responsible for direct inflammatory effects, while also stimulating appetite." Digestion of wheat works like this: When digested by stomach acids and enzymes, the gliadin becomes an exorphin, a morphine-like compound, which binds to opiate receptors in your brain. These exorphins, however, don't relieve pain like other opiates; instead, they cause addictive behavior and appetite stimulation that can result in the consumption of more than four hundred additional calories every day! Dr. Davis asserts that modern wheat is as addictive as many drugs. The purveyors of wheat-based foods act as unwitting local drug dealers, supplying another hit of obesity-inducing exorphins before you can say "gluten."

And speaking of gluten . . . wheat also contains gluten, something many of us have now either heard of or may have seen mentioned in the media as a Poor Food. It is generally accepted that one in 133 people have celiac disease, a genetic condition resulting in intestinal damage whenever a sufferer ingests gluten. However, many medical and nutritional experts believe that the number of people with undiagnosed gluten sensitivity is potentially much higher, perhaps as high as 30 to 50 percent of the entire population! Sensitivity to gluten causes digestive problems, headaches, eczema-like skin symptoms, brain fog, and fatigue. Dr. Davis says, "The gluten protein is responsible for the destructive inflammatory effects on bowel and central nervous system health."

The negative effects of gluten might not be readily apparent to you, and you have likely come to tolerate them over the course of your lifetime. Millions of people around the world have eliminated gluten from their diets and have reported an elimination of subclinical symptoms of poor health they didn't even realize they had! Bloating and gas after meals disappearing, brain fog that hit every afternoon suddenly lifting, going from several mild colds each year to zero for years, dramatic improvements in acne conditions without drugs, elimination of migraines, and much more!

There are two other compounds occurring in wheat that Dr. Davis also warns against—lectins and amylopectin A. "The lectins in wheat likely underlie the increased intestinal permeability to multiple foreign proteins that cascade into inflammatory and autoimmune conditions like rheumatoid arthritis and lupus. The amylopectin A is responsible for the expansion of visceral fat [unhealthy fat that surrounds the organs] in the abdomen, the 'wheat belly' that in turn leads to inflammation, insulin resistance, diabetes, arthritis, and heart disease." (It is this amylopectin A that is responsible for the high blood sugar spike caused by eating wheat.)

So the bottom line is that you really don't need wheat, and eliminating wheat from your diet will result in numerous health benefits. By cutting out wheat, you may just save yourself from a variety of health conditions, including intestinal disease, inflammation, arthritis, acid reflux, indigestion, schizophrenia, leg swelling and numbness, brain fog, obesity, insulin resistance, heart disease, diabetes, behavioral outbursts in children with ADHD, addiction, allergies, high blood sugar, adverse cholesterol values, and more.

Kamut and Spelt

While arguably better choices than "wheat," these two grains are actually ancient ancestors of modern-day wheat and are therefore still considered undesirable in the long run. Both grains still contain gliadins (although they have lower potent appetite stimulation than modern wheat) as well as gluten and lectins. We recommend steering clear of these ancient grains often named on specialty boxed cereals, breads, and pastas, as they both increase blood sugar—exactly the opposite of what modern nutritional science recommends for optimal health.

Oats, Rice, Corn (GMO Alert), Buckwheat, Quinoa, Millet, and Amaranth

These gluten-free grains (note: buckwheat, quinoa, millet, and amaranth are technically seeds) do not contain many of the problematic compounds of wheat that we have just discussed. But because they are high in carbohydrates, they still increase blood sugar, which can lead to insulin resistance and a host of other related health problems.

These grains, like wheat, also contain the Everyday Micronutrient Depleter, phytic acid, an acid we discussed in *Naked Calories* that binds to and blocks the absorption of calcium, magnesium, copper, manganese, chromium, iron, zinc, and niacin and accelerates the metabolism of vitamin D, causing depletion of this important anti-obesity vitamin. Soaking, sprouting, or souring these grains will reduce their phytic acid content, but it will not eliminate it entirely.

Due to the new understanding of the dangers of wheat, millet is now manufactured as the go-to wheat substitute. However, it is perhaps the most goitrogenic food in the world. Remember, goitrogens are substances that hinder the uptake of iodine, which causes suppressed thyroid function. This means that substituting millet for wheat makes you susceptible to iodine deficiency, causing thyroid problems that can lead to lowered metabolism. If you decide to make millet one of your food

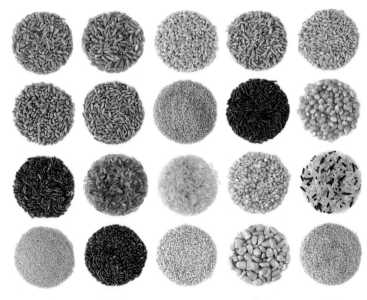

choices, consider an iodine supplement, or eat iodine-rich seafood (see Aisle 3: Fish and Seafood) and/or seaweed snacks (see Aisle 8: Snacks). Additionally, another one of these psuedo-grain options, quinoa, has gut-irritating and inflammatory side effects due to its content of soap-like molecules called saponins. While rinsing quinoa can be helpful, many individuals with gluten sensitivity find themselves similarly affected after eating quinoa.

And don't forget about arsenic! According to a November 2012 report by *Consumer Reports,* arsenic levels in many brands of rice (brown more than white)—as well as popular rice products like baby formulas, rice pastas, rice syrups, and rice-based cereals—are at worrisome and potentially dangerous levels. With so many people now choosing gluten-free foods, rice consumption has increased, and with it, exposure to both inorganic arsenic (a carcinogen) and organic arsenic (less toxic, but still a concern). To reduce your exposure, scientists at *Consumer Reports* recommend restricting rice and rice-based hot cereal, ready-to-eat cereal, rice pasta, and rice cakes to two to three servings a week for adults and one to one-and-a-half servings a week for children. (To learn more, go to NotInMyFood.org.)

If you still want grains in your diet, these gluten-free grains are your best bet. Regardless of the grain you eat, we advise you to use them sparingly, and always soak, sprout, or sour your grains when possible to reduce phytic acid and enhance micronutrient absorption.

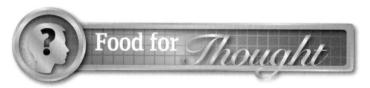

Have you ever wondered how the Os in Cheerios are made or how macaroni is formed into cute, hollow, bite-sized elbows, wagon wheels, or letter shapes? Well, it is done through a manufacturing process known as extrusion. Extrusion is the act of taking a preconditioned mix and passing it through an extruder (long tube) where it is then forced through a die, molded to its desired shape, and cut to the desired length. The problem is that a lot of heat is given off during this process, which, just as pasteurization and homogenization denatures the protein and fatty acids in dairy products, damages the protein and starch structure of many cold cereals, pastas, premade cookie dough, some French fries, certain baby foods, ready-to-eat snacks, and dry and semi-moist pet food. So, while extrusion makes the ABCs in alphabet soup cute, they may not be as smart as we once thought.

Now that we understand the nature of wheat, and many of the other grains on the market, we can safely push our cart through the supermarket to examine the extensive list of grain-filled products. We'll start with the cereal aisle because, after all, that is the food with which many people start their day.

GRAINS

Cereal

With the new information you have just learned about grains, it is time to look at the boxes of cereal in a whole new light. Here is the ingredient list of a typical cereal you might buy for your family—Post Select Blueberry Morning. (We didn't opt to review a children's sugar-coated cereal because many of you already purchase healthier options.) Post recently upgraded this cereal by removing the partially hydrogenated oil (aka trans fats) it used to contain, so we figured it was fair game. After all, they have obviously recently reviewed their own ingredients and deemed them a healthy start to your day.

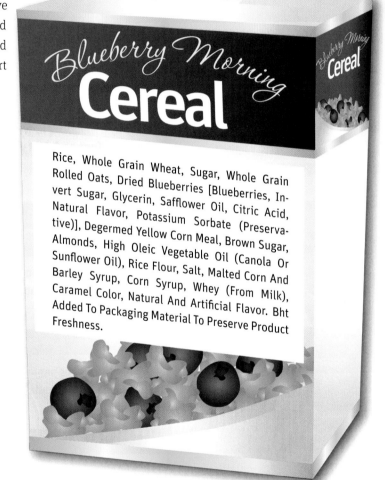

Rice, Whole Grain Wheat, Sugar, Whole Grain Rolled Oats, Dried Blueberries [Blueberries, Invert Sugar, Glycerin, Safflower Oil, Citric Acid, Natural Flavor, Potassium Sorbate (Preservative)], Degermed Yellow Corn Meal, Brown Sugar, Almonds, High Oleic Vegetable Oil (Canola Or Sunflower Oil), Rice Flour, Salt, Malted Corn And Barley Syrup, Corn Syrup, Whey (From Milk), Caramel Color, Natural And Artificial Flavor. Bht Added To Packaging Material To Preserve Product Freshness.

Wow, now that is a *lot* of ingredients in one serving of cereal! Remember, the grains and sugars are all carbohydrates, and your body converts all forms of carbohydrates into glucose when you ingest them. Every time sugar and carbohydrates appear on the label, you should recognize that they will increase your blood sugar, which leads to weight gain, insulin resistance, diabetes, and a host of other health conditions. So, let's revisit this ingredient list using our handy sugar decoder.

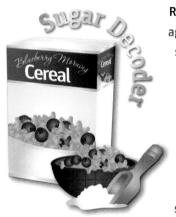

Rice (sugar-induced insulin spike), **Whole Grain Wheat** (sugar again), **Sugar** (GMO and EMD), **Whole Grain Rolled Oats** (still sugar), **Dried Blueberry(ies)** (more sugar), **Invert Sugar** (more GMO sugar), **Glycerin** (sugar substitute), **Safflower Oil, Citric Acid** (GMO), **Natural Flavor(s), Potassium Sorbate** (Preservative), **Degermed Yellow Corn Meal** (more GMO sugar), **Brown Sugar** (sugar of another color), **Almond(s), Vegetable(s) Oil High Oleic (Canola** (GMO) **or Sunflower Oil), Rice Flour** (still sugar), **Salt, Malted Corn** (GMO sugar) **and Malted Barley Syrup** (GMO syrupy sugar) **Corn Syrup** (more GMO syrup), **Whey from Milk** (possible rBGH), **Caramel Color** (possible carcinogen), **Flavoring Artificial And Natural** (MSG), **Bht Added To Preserve Freshness** (possible carcinogen).

Now do you see just how much sugar is really being delivered by this "healthy" cereal? So, how much sugar are you really eating? In one single serving, a small bowl at best, you're getting 16 grams of sugar. That is more than eight sugar-filled candy Pixy Stix. Would you even consider having that for breakfast? Or feeding it to a child? And that doesn't even consider the grains that will also spike your insulin. Sixteen grams represents only the added sugar content. And how would this satiate you? Would it supply the protein or fat calories needed to reduce hunger and lower your daily caloric intake? Not likely. This cereal supplies a mere three grams of protein—less than half the protein in one egg. Protein and fat take longer for the body to digest than unhealthier sources of processed food, helping to keep hunger pangs at bay. All you would get from this bowl of cereal is a sugar rush, followed by a catastrophic energy crash, followed by a craving for more sugar.

Building a Better Breakfast

We've all heard that breakfast is the most important meal of the day, and recent studies have now solidified that motto. According to scientists from the University of Missouri, breakfast-skippers tend to weigh more and have other unhealthy habits. But you may be surprised that it wasn't the act of eating breakfast alone that determined the benefit, but *what* participants ate for breakfast that ultimately proved to be the most important factor. Only individuals who ate high-protein breakfasts reported more satiety and less overeating throughout the day.

The study, which used magnetic imaging of the brain, concluded that a protein-rich breakfast reduces brain signals that control food desires and cravings, even several hours after eating. According to research by Donald Layman, PhD, of the University of Illinois, individuals who start the day with a protein-rich breakfast consume two hundred fewer calories a day than those who chow down on a carb-heavy breakfast like cereal or bagels.

GRAINS

The breakfast of our grandparents or great-grandparents prior to the explosion of modern packaged foods was free from processed carbs and likely centered on nutritious protein- and fat-based foods, such as sliced meat, bacon, some eggs, milk, and perhaps cheese. Today, most people don't find time to sit down for a proper breakfast. They rely on quick-and-easy, high-carb, insulin-spiking options such as bagels, breakfast pockets, breakfast bars, scones, muffins. We urge you to wake a few minutes earlier to prepare a meal that will gear you up for the rest of your day and ready your child for a positive learning experience.

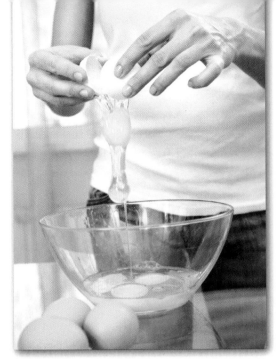

This is why we prefer our clients not eat cereal at all and opt for more traditional breakfasts—the ones our grandparents used to eat. But if you just aren't ready to ditch your morning bowl of milk and grain, check out our choices for some of the best cereal swaps below in our Steer Here section. These boxed breakfasts use better grain options with no added sugars. But first . . .

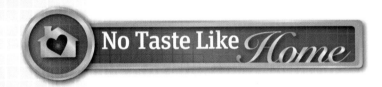

How can you find the time to cook a healthy egg-enhanced breakfast every morning? You don't have to. This tasty shortcut stores in the fridge or freezer and makes a great grab-and-go breakfast. Lose the wheat-filled muffin . . . save the muffin tin. Enjoy egg muffins to load up on your protein and fill your body with a fresh array of delicious micronutrient-rich vegetables.

Protein-Packed Morning Muffins

INGREDIENTS

- 5 large pastured eggs
- ¼ cup organic sour cream (you choose the fat content)
- Unrefined sea salt and organic pepper to taste
- Organic cayenne pepper to taste (boost metabolism all day long; see page 219)
- ⅔ cup freshly chopped or grated organic cheese, or cheese combo of your choice
- ⅓ organic tomato, chopped
- 1 chopped garlic (let sit for ten minutes prior to cooking; see page 141)
- ⅓ onion (it's on the Fab Fourteen, so save money by purchasing non-organic)
- ⅓ cup cooked organic spinach or asparagus
- 6 slices of pastured, sodium nitrate–free bacon

DIRECTIONS

1. Preheat oven to 325 degrees.

2. Grease a muffin tin with ghee, coconut oil, butter, or retained and collected fat, or use a nonstick tin. You will use only six of the muffin molds (perhaps seven depending on the bulk of vegetables and bacon).

3. Brown bacon and chop. Use the remaining bacon fat to cook onion and garlic until onion is translucent.

4. Beat eggs in a small bowl and blend with sour cream, grated cheese, and desired organic seasonings.

5. Pour egg mixture into six muffin molds until two-thirds full, keeping enough room on top for bacon and/or vegetables.

6. Mix vegetables and bacon in the now-empty egg bowl, and distribute evenly into the egg mixture.

7. Bake for approximately 25 minutes or until cooked through. Allow to completely cool before removing from muffin tin.

You can also use this recipe for leftovers. Imagine chopping up your chicken breast with a few broccoli spears and cheddar cheese. How about the burger no one finished and some blue cheese? The combinations are endless, and you save money while delivering a breakfast fit for a king (even a busy king, or queen, on the run).

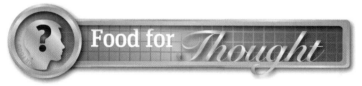

Food for Thought

Not an egg eater but still in search of a great protein-enriched breakfast? Here are a few other great options to make sure you make the most of your morning meal.

1 GREEK YOGURT. Top 1 cup of organic Greek yogurt with fresh organic berries and sprouted seeds or nuts (see page 64). Adding organic berries delivers great anti-oxidants while the sprouted nuts/seeds can add healthy fats that support satiety.

2 IT'S TIME TO BETTER YOUR BURGER. Yes, burgers don't have to be limited to lunch and dinner. Enjoy mini burger bites with eggs. You can pan grill a couple grass-fed ground beef burgers or ground pastured chicken/turkey patties, and enjoy them with fried eggs on top. Skip the bun—allow the meat to sop up the yolk.

3 LEARN YOUR WAY FROM NORWAY. The Vikings had it right when they created their traditional breakfast of wild-caught smoked salmon. Our pinwheel recipe (see page 123) makes a protein-packed treat that you can enjoy with your fingers and can prepare the night before.

GRAINS

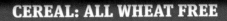
CEREAL: ALL WHEAT FREE

LYDIA'S ORGANICS SPROUTED CINNAMON CEREAL

- Organic
- Sprouted seeds and nuts
- Sweetener free

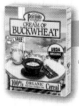

LOUISE'S GRAIN-FREE GRANOLA OR BREAKFAST BITES

- Coconut flour (think MCT)
- Chia (think omega-3)
- Sweetened with stevia
- Delicious cinnamon taste

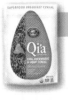

NATURE'S PATH QI'A SUPERFOOD (ORIGINAL FLAVOR)

- Organic
- Chia and hemp (seeds high in omega-3s)
- Buckwheat (a seed, not a grain)

ANCIENT QUINOA HARVEST QUINOA FLAKES

- Organic
- Quinoa is a good source of protein

POCONO BRAND CREAM OF BUCKWHEAT

- Organic
- Buckwheat
- Cooks in ninety seconds

STEER CLEAR

CEREAL

POST MARSHMALLOW PEBBLES

Your child will be bouncing off the walls when he gets to school. Not only will the four artificial colors kill his concentration, but a fifth color, caramel color, may be carcinogenic. The many denatured protein shapes are filled with GMO sugars, trans fats, and BHT. If the artificial colors don't cause your child to be hyperactive, the 10 grams of sugar most certainly will.

ALBERTSON'S LOW-FAT GRANOLA RAISIN BRAN

Granola is a health food, right? With seven forms of added sugar (sugar, high fructose corn syrup, brown sugar, corn syrup, barley malt syrup, glycine, and honey) and four insulin-spiking grains (wheat, rice, wheat bran, and oats), you'll be packing on the pounds before you make it to lunch. A one-cup serving is equal to five packets of sugar. Coat these GMO crunchy bits with trans fats and possible carcinogens (BHT), and you're so not setting the stage for a successful day.

❑ Choose other breakfast options over cereal.

❑ Choose high-protein breakfasts.

❑ Choose low sugar content.

❑ Choose buckwheat, quinoa, millet, flax, hemp, and amaranth.

❑ Choose organic.

❑ Avoid GMO corn and corn sugars.

❑ Avoid wheat.

*My go-to Rich Food choices for cereal:*_____

_____

_____

_____

_____

_____

_____

_____

Bread: America's Favorite JUNK Food

We now know that wheat, the main ingredient in bread, is addictive. The more we eat it, the more we need to eat it. But it is not just the wheat in bread that is hurting us. Bread often contains a host of other Poor Food ingredients as well. Let's take a closer look.

Top 10 Poor Food Ingredients in Bread

1 All wheat, even whole grain or sprouted, contains gliadin, gluten, lectins, and amylopectin A.

2 Sugar and Sinister Sugar Substitutes, including high fructose corn syrup, dextrose, maltodextrin, aspartame, sucralose, honey, evaporated cane sugar, and agave nectar.

3 Trans fats, including partially hydrogenated oils and mono and diglycerides.

4 Soybean oil and/or canola oil (GMO alert).

5 MSG (Criminal Chameleon) under its numerous obesity-inducing aliases.

6 Potassium bromate—potentially carcinogenic iodine thieving Banned Bad Boy (BBB).

7 Azodicarbonamide—asthma-inducing Banned Bad Boy (BBB).

8 Soy lecithin (GMO alert).

9 DATEM (Diacetyl Tartaric Acid Esters of Monoglycerides). Another dough conditioner used to improve volume and uniformity. It is considered safe by the FDA, but a 2002 study on rats showed "heart muscle fibrosis and adrenal overgrowth."

10 Artificial colors and preservatives (including the likely carcinogens BHA and BHT).

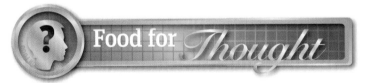

Food for *Thought*

If you think about it, bread is just a delivery system for other, more nutritious foods like meats and cheeses. After all, the grains are processed and stripped of their micronutrients. So, wouldn't it make sense to consider a different delivery system, perhaps one with fewer *naked calories?* Why not try a lettuce wrap? Not only are they really trendy, popping up on numerous restaurant menus, but they are easy to make, and you can use just about anything you may have left over from the night before. You don't have to lose any of the convenience of the grab-and-go sandwich, either. Choose lettuce with big leaves such as iceberg, romaine, or red leaf to create the sturdiest wraps. Don't forget, because lettuce is one of the Terrible Twenty, choose organic when possible.

Here are three great lettuce wrap options to satisfy everyone in the family.

1 THE CLUB Turkey, bacon, shredded lettuce and tomato.

2 TACO SALAD Grass-fed ground beef with organic taco seasonings, freshly shredded cheese, avocado, and salsa. Add a side of sour cream for dipping!

3 THE ROMAN Grilled chicken, cheese, chopped cucumber, and tomatoes in homemade Caesar salad dressing (see recipe, page 163).

*Always use the best Rich Food ingredients.

Lusting over a loaf of bread? Or fancy French toast? You can satisfy your urge while still not giving in to grains. Make this simple fifteen-minute recipe and curb your cravings.

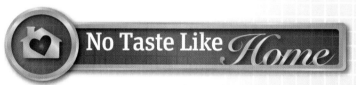

By avoiding wheat altogether, your addiction to it will soon pass.

The Caltons' No-Belly Bread

INGREDIENTS

- ¼ cup extra virgin organic coconut oil (melted)
- ⅛ cup organic almond flour
- ⅛ cup coconut flour
- ¼ cup unflavored whey protein
- 5 large pastured eggs

- ½ tsp. unrefined sea salt
- 1 tsp. baking powder (look for one that is aluminum free)
- (Not familiar with these fantastic flours? Read more about them in Aisle 7: Baking.)

DIRECTIONS

 1 Preheat oven to 375 degrees.

2 Mix in ingredients, and whisk until smooth.

 3 Spread thin on a greased baking sheet, and cut rectangular slices or purchase a doughnut pan to create homemade no-belly bagels. The shape may be different, but the recipe remains the same.

 4 Bake for 15 minutes.

OPTION 1: *Swirl in a mixture of cinnamon and powdered pure stevia or alternative sugar substitute to create delicious cinnamon bread.*

OPTION 2: *Add in freshly grated Parmesan cheese and garlic powder for a zesty, savory Italian splurge.*

OPTION 3: *Take the baking sheet "sliced bread" and dip in egg batter for a delicious French toast (see Aisle 5: Condiments for Rich Food syrup options).*

Want to see just how many options are out there? Just head on over to the Rich Food Resource Center and watch the step-by-step No-Belly Bread recipe tutorial.

GRAINS

WHILE OUR TOP PICK is to skip the bread aisle altogether and opt to make *The Caltons' No-Belly Bread*, here are our choices for the best options on the market.

BREAD

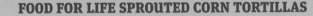

Coupon Clipper

FOOD FOR LIFE SPROUTED CORN TORTILLAS

- Organic sprouted whole kernel corn
- Wheat free
- Sugar free

LYDIA'S ORGANICS SUNFLOWER SEED BREAD

- Organic
- Sprouted
- Wheat free
- Sugar free

SAMI'S BAKERY MILLET AND FLAX BREAD AND PIZZA CRUST

- Organic
- Wheat free
- High omega-3
- Sugar free

SAMI'S BAKERY MILLET BANANA BREAD

- Organic
- Wheat free
- Sugar free

DELAND BAKERY MILLET BREAD

- Organic
- Wheat free
- Sugar free

STEER CLEAR

BREAD

SCHWEBEL'S CINNABON CINNAMON BREAD

This bread has twenty-two Poor Food ingredients that can be found in 9 out of our 10 Reasons Not to Eat Bread list: 1. wheat flour, vital wheat gluten, bleached wheat flour, 2. sugar, brown sugar, fructose, raisin juice concentrate, dextrose, acesulfame potassium, 3. hydrogenated soybean and/or cottonseed oil, mono-glycerides, 4. soybean oil, 5. natural flavors, natural and artificial flavors (again), enzymes, 6. malt barley flour, 7. azodicarbonamide, 8. soy lecithin, 9. amazingly does not contain DATEM, 10. BHA, caramel color, red #40. On their website, the Schwebel family pledges to provide you and your family with fresh, wholesome, nutritious, and great-tasting bread products. We pledge to inform you that these cinnabons are a sinful mess.

WONDER BREAD SMART WHEAT

It's a *wonder* anyone buys this stuff. There is nothing smart about eating the wheat, sugar (EMD), added wheat gluten, soybean oil (GMO), mono and diglycerides (trans fats), soybean oil (GMO), cottonseed fiber (GMO), soy lecithin (GMO), and azodicarbonamide (BBB) in this loaf. Eat this, and you may *wonder* where your toes went (hint: Your waistline is now obscuring your view).

☐ Choose lettuce for wraps.

☐ Choose wheat-free options.

☐ Avoid breads that contain ingredients on the Top 10 Ingredients in Bread to Avoid list.

My go-to Rich Food choices for breads: _____

_____

_____

_____

_____

_____

_____

_____

_____

_____

_____

_____

_____

Checkout Checklist

Pasta

From penne primavera to baked ziti to your little one's mac and cheese, the shapes and sizes may change, but the factors you must consider when choosing the nicest noodles for your next meal remain the same.

We have already reviewed the different grains available and discussed which ones might be the best digested and healthiest for your body. We have explained that wheat contains compounds that can cause increased appetite, behavioral outbursts in children with ADHD, dementia, and a drug-like food addiction. However, if you still desire a rigatoni for your red sauce and aren't ready to break the grain addiction, we have highlighted a few of the best options available. But first . . .

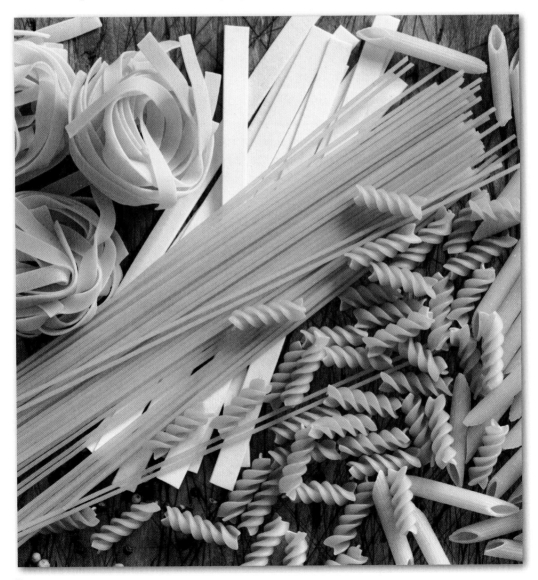

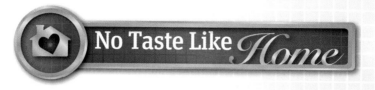

No Taste Like *Home*

Nix the noodles, and save yourself a grain-loaded gut! Try this simple macaroni makeover. Replace your store-bought spaghetti with this zucchini spaghetti dish (we call it zughetti) and save yourself more than 400 calories per three-cup micronutrient-rich serving. (See our Rich Food, Poor Food head-to-head comparison below for more great reasons to give this recipe a chance.)

Zughetti Macaroni Makeover

INGREDIENTS

- Organic Zucchini (approximately 2 zucchinis per person)
- Unrefined sea salt
- Rich Food sauce of your choice

DIRECTIONS

 1 Prepare the zucchini into noodles using either an inexpensive julienne peeler or vegetable mandolin/spiral slicer. You can find our favorite picks in the Rich Food Resource Center at CaltonNutrition.com. We love the long zughetti ribbons that the slicer forms—you can even wrap them around a fork like the real thing! This incredible kitchen gadget can also be used to slice your veggie chips (see recipe, page 231) and only costs around thirty dollars—a small investment with a ton of great uses.

 2 Put the zughetti ribbons in a colander, and toss in with two teaspoons of unrefined sea salt. The salt with help pull the water out of the zucchini and make them even more noodle-like. Place the colander over a bowl to catch released water. Let stand for twenty minutes.

 3 Rinse the zughetti well.

 4 Place the rinsed zughetti in a pot of boiling water for one minute to cook. Rinse immediately with cold water to stop cooking.

5 Place in a serving bowl and cover with your sauce.

Not convinced? We'll show you how to create a perfect zughetti dinner online in the Rich Food Resource Center video database.

GRAINS

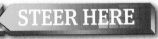

STEER HERE

PASTA

OUR TOP PICK! Zughetti-Macaroni Makeover
- Grain free   • Just as hearty

EDEN ORGANIC SOBA 100% BUCKWHEAT

- Organic   • Buckwheat (non-grain) source (100 percent)   • Gluten free

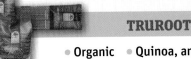

TRUROOTS ANCIENT GRAINS PASTA

- Organic   • Quinoa, amaranth, and brown rice   • Gluten free

TINYADA ORGANIC BROWN RICE PASTA

- Organic   • Brown rice (fairly low in reported arsenic)   • Gluten free

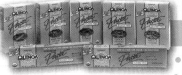

ANCIENT QUINOA HARVEST PASTAS

- Organic   • Non-GMO corn flour   • Quinoa flour
- Gluten free

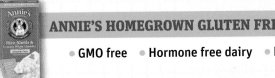

ANNIE'S HOMEGROWN GLUTEN FREE RICE PASTA & CHEDDAR

- GMO free   • Hormone free dairy   • Rice flour   • Gluten free

MIRACLE NOODLE SHIRATAKI PASTA

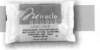

- Low calorie   • Gluten free

This nearly tasteless, traditional Japanese noodle is made from a highly fibrous konjac root. They are a great way to soak up some sauce without adding in wheat or carbohydrates.

PASTA

PASTA RONI PARMESAN CHEESE

The famous makers of Rice-A-Roni begin with wheat flour (think refined, belly-bloating, gluten-gut nightmare) and top it with GMO corn syrup, hormone-filled dairy, MSG under three different aliases, and three artificial colors to help make these ingredients look more natural than they are. San Francisco treat? More like trick!

KRAFT EASY MAC, MACARONI & CHEESE SINGLE SERVING MICROWAVE BOWL

This classic children's favorite serves up a whopping 440 calories of yuck! The wheat flour (aka refined white flour, EMD) is coated with a gooey combination of corn syrup solids (sugar-based GMO), maltodextrin (MSG, GMO), artificial flavors (MSG), two artificial colors, guar gum (EMD), and monosodium glutamate (obesity inducing).

Pasta Sauce

PRIMAVERA, PUTTANESCA, OR PESTO . . . Regardless of preference, you can add in a lot of unwanted Poor Food ingredients if you don't read labels carefully. When shopping in this aisle, make sure to be on the lookout for added sugars, GMOs, and MSG under numerous aliases. Some smart sauce makers even know to package in opaque jars to lock in micronutrients.

GRAINS

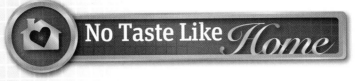
No Taste Like *Home*

While there is nothing wrong with our Steer Here pasta sauce picks, why not try these two simple sauces you can make in less than fifteen minutes? These sauces aren't just for noodles or zughetti—enjoy them over your favorite meat, chicken, and seafood dishes.

Rich & Creamy Alfredo

INGREDIENTS

- 4 Tbsp. unsalted organic grass-fed butter
- ⅔ cup freshly grated organic Parmesan cheese
- ½ cup organic grass-fed heavy cream (preferably unpasteurized)
- 1 large pasture-raised organic egg
- Organic black pepper to taste
- 1 garlic clove, cut 10 minutes prior to heating (see page 141)

DIRECTIONS

 1 Melt butter in a sauté pan over low heat.

 2 Add in egg and cream and combine, raising heat to medium.

 3 Add in garlic and slowly add in cheese while stirring so as not to clump.

 4 When fully combined, season with black pepper.

Add in portobello mushrooms for an earthy, meat-like quality.

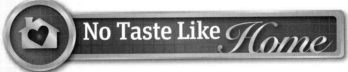
No Taste Like *Home*

Perfect Pesto

INGREDIENTS

- 2 cups packed fresh organic basil leaves
- ½ cup freshly grated organic Parmesan or Romano cheese
- ¼ cup organic pine nuts
- 2 large garlic cloves, quartered
- Unrefined sea salt to taste
- ¼ cup cold-pressed organic extra virgin olive oil

DIRECTIONS

1 Combine basil, cheese, pine nuts, and garlic into a food processor and blend until evenly and finely chopped.

 2 On a low setting, slowly add olive oil until the sauce has a thick, even texture.

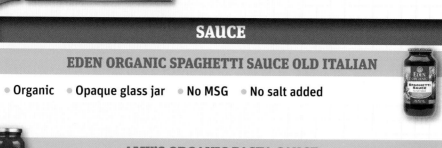

SAUCE

EDEN ORGANIC SPAGHETTI SAUCE OLD ITALIAN

- Organic - Opaque glass jar - No MSG - No salt added

AMY'S ORGANIC PASTA SAUCE

- Organic - No MSG

MOM'S ORGANIC TRADITIONAL PASTA SAUCE

- Organic - No MSG   Also try their organic roasted pepper sauce

MARIO BATALI ALFREDO SAUCE

- No sugar added

STEER CLEAR

SAUCE

CLASSICO ROASTED RED PEPPER ALFREDO SAUCE

Imagine a big pot of non-organic cream, butter, and cheese (synthetic hormones and antibiotics), red peppers (Terrible Twenty), enzyme modified egg yolks (MSG), modified cornstarch (GMO, MSG), sugar (EMD), irradiated black pepper (EMD), high maltose corn syrup solids (GMO), and soybean oil (GMO) simmering on the stove. Sound appetizing?

MOM'S MARTINI PASTA SAUCE

While Mom's got our Steer Here pick for the organic traditional pasta sauce (which we love!), Mom's gets our Steer Clear pick here because the sauce contains sugar (an EMD ingredient in the stock), yeast extract (MSG), maltodextrin (sugar), soybeans (GMO), modified food starch (GMO, MSG), guar gum (EMD), carrageenan (possible carcinogen, MSG), and loads of non-organic spices (EMD). This is a good example of how companies who are doing the right thing with some of their products still need to improve with others. Read labels carefully before buying even trusted brands, and don't be afraid to sound off as a consumer. Most companies have website contact forms or consumer hotlines where you can let them know how you feel about their products, good and bad. If we all chime in, consumer pressure can and will lead to real change in the grocery store!

Checkout Checklist

☐ Choose zughetti for a hearty and healthy pasta substitute.

☐ Choose organic pasta that is wheat free.

☐ Choose organic tomato sauce.

☐ Choose pasta sauce in opaque glass jars.

☐ Choose to cook your own quick pasta sauces that are versatile with meat, chicken, and seafood fare as well.

☐ Avoid pasta sauce that contains sugar.

☐ Avoid pasta sauce with non-organic irradiated spices.

My go-to Rich Food choices for pasta and sauces: _____

_____

_____

_____

_____

_____

_____

_____

_____

RICH FOOD vs POOR FOOD

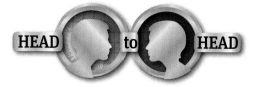

2 cups of Zughetti with 1 cup of
Eden Organic Spaghetti Sauce
Old Italian

2 cups of Barilla Spaghetti
with 1 cup of Mom's Martini
Pasta Sauce

180	Calories	620
300 percent more! A whopping 28 grams	Lycopene	Lacking due to non-organic tomatoes
Organic	Spices	Irradiated (EMD)
None added	GMO ingredients	Soybeans and modified cornstarch
None added	Sugar	Sugar and maltodextrin added
None added	MSG	Modified cornstarch and yeast extract
Wheat free	Grains	Refined white flour

Remember: We aren't trying to limit your calories, but this low-calorie recipe saves room for a micronutrient-rich appetizer and dessert.

Fewer micronutrients; more EMDs, GMOs, and sugars; and will cause over-eating, bloating, and leaky gut.

Rice & Beans

It is time to make over the Mexican fiesta and do over bean dips. Much like the other food swaps we discussed in the grains category, your belly will be all the better with Rich Food versions.

. . . .

Rice

WE ALREADY INCLUDED RICE in our "better grain if you're going to eat grain" category, but we want to say a little more on this topic because choosing the right rice is a bit paradoxical. What do we mean? Well, we all have heard that brown rice or wild rice is more micronutrient packed than refined white rice—and therefore theoretically better to eat. However, brown rice and wild rice also contain phytic acid—a potent Everyday Micronutrient Depleter (EMD). So, what to do? We really only have two options. We can soak/ferment brown or wild rice with a somewhat laborious but highly effective process (detailed shortly), or we can eat refined white rice. If we have planned ahead at least a day, we can exercise the first option. But here is the paradox: if you are out at a restaurant or dining at a friend's house and there is a choice between brown/wild rice (not soaked/fermented) and white rice, you would be better off eating the refined white rice because of its lack of phytic acid. Make no mistake, the white rice will not contribute to your micronutrient sufficiency, but it will not deplete it to any great extent, either.

So, except for the blood sugar spike, and the potential allergic reactions some people can get from rice (especially those with wheat sensitivities), the white rice is a benign meal filler. Well, benign unless you are carrying unwanted body fat. In which case, our tendency to fill meals with grain-based carbohydrate foods can be the difference between effortlessly maintaining our ideal body composition over decades or falling into the statistical average that an American gains 1.5 pounds of fat each year from age twenty-five to fifty-five (and loses a half-pound of muscle each year).

When you center your diet around Rich Foods with high micronutrient values, you will gain a greater sense of satiety from your meals and snacks and naturally regulate your caloric intake without the usual struggling and suffering. By all means, make the best choices with your rice, pasta, or bread products, but remember that opting out is also a choice!

Regardless of the shade of rice you choose, purchasing only organic rice will save you from the thirteen known pesticides commonly found in conventional rice. Remember, recent reports also show rice to have high levels of arsenic. Thoroughly rinsing and cooking your rice with six cups of water to one cup of rice and then draining the excess water is one way to reduce this harmful carcinogen. While this will lead to more micro-nutrient loss than conventional methods of cooking, it can reduce inorganic arsenic content by about 30 percent.

Looking for a way to prepare whole brown rice that increases its mineral availability? Well, look no further. Neurobiologist Dr. Stephan Guyenet discovered an effective way to ferment rice and beans and reduce phytic acid by up to 96 percent! Based on a scientific paper out of Beijing that studied the effects of soaking, sprouting, and fermentation on phytic acid in brown rice, Dr. Guyenet noted that researchers found it was the fermentation process and not the soaking that effectively degraded phytic acid—even better than sprouting. Here is a traditional Chinese proce-dure for fermenting brown rice.

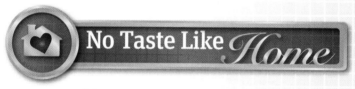

Chinese Fermented Brown Rice

DIRECTIONS

 1 Soak brown rice in *dechlorinated (filtered)* water for 24 hours at room temperature without changing the water.

 2 Reserve 10 percent of the soaking liquid (Liquid A), which has a good refrigerated shelf life.

 3 Discard the remainder of soaking liquid.

 4 Cook the rice in fresh water. (Al-though the phytic acid has been reduced in this first batch, it is still higher than we would like.)

 5 The next time you make brown rice, add the soaking liquid you reserved from the last batch (Liquid A) to the new soaking water at the beginning of the soaking process. (This batch of brown rice will contain less phytic acid than the first.)

 6 Repeat the cycle. The process will gradually improve until 96 percent or more of the phytic acid is de-graded.

By the third batch, better rice is revealed! This same fermentation process is great for other grains and beans as well.

GRAINS

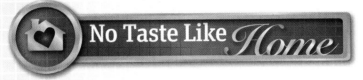

As we stated earlier, sometimes it is best to opt out of starchy carbohydrates. On those occasions, we serve our Rockin' Rice Replacement. Our guests just love this versatile recipe. Don't be shy—get creative! Add in curry spices for Indian-inspired rice or stir-fry in assorted vegetables for traditional Asian fried rice. This rockin' remix replaces the rice with cauliflower. It's a quick fix that gives you all the satisfaction with none of the waistline growing action.

Rockin' Rice Replacement

INGREDIENTS:

- 1 head of cauliflower (not on Terrible Twenty)
- 2 tbsp. organic coconut oil. You can substitute a high-quality Rich Food butter or ghee if preferred.
- Customize with organic seasonings of choice

DIRECTIONS:

1 Chop cauliflower until it reaches a rice-like consistency. This is easiest in a food processor. Do not over-process.

2 In a skillet, sauté the diced cauliflower in the melted coconut oil for approximately five minutes until the cauliflower begins to soften.

3 Season the rice to create an endless amount of options.

Beans

WHILE BEANS ARE WILDLY POPULAR around the world (black beans in Latin America or chickpeas in the Middle East), they contain food components—many of the same found in grains—that can strip away essential minerals, cause digestive disorders, and lead to obesity and diabetes by spiking your insulin with a heavy load of carbohydrates.

Legumes contain phytic acid, which inhibits micronutrient absorption. Like wheat and other grains, beans contain lectins, which, when digested, cause your body to produce antibodies, triggering autoimmune issues, including type 1 diabetes, celiac disease, lupus, and multiple sclerosis. To make matters worse, lectins damage the walls of your intestines, contributing to "leaky gut," a condition that can be the precipice of food allergies. While the lectin concerns with beans is less than that of grains, and thus these foods are less objectionable in the diet than grains, lectin ingestion might still be a major concern for folks with sensitive digestive systems. Finally, beans are high in carbohydrates, and when you eat them, they break down to sugar—spiking your insulin and sending you one step closer to weight gain, insulin resistance, and type 2 diabetes.

Now, for those individuals who still want beans, perhaps for their protein or fiber content, we can't avoid the insulin spike, but we can greatly reduce levels of phytic acid and lectins through a soaking, sprouting, and fermenting process. Follow the guidelines for fermenting rice in *There's No Taste Like Home* mentioned previously.

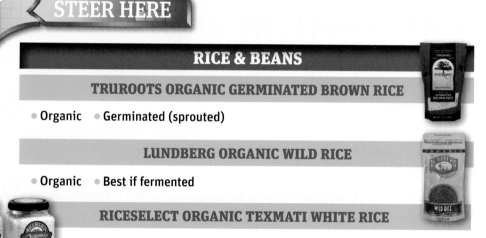

STEER HERE

RICE & BEANS

TRUROOTS ORGANIC GERMINATED BROWN RICE

- Organic • Germinated (sprouted)

LUNDBERG ORGANIC WILD RICE

- Organic • Best if fermented

RICESELECT ORGANIC TEXMATI WHITE RICE

- Organic • Choose if not fermenting
Also try their organic brown rice (best if fermented)

TRUROOTS ORGANIC SPROUTED QUINOA

- Organic • Sprouted • High in protein
- Cooks in just fifteen minutes (stovetop) *Also try their Organic Sprouted Bean Trio.*

EDEN ORGANIC REFRIED PINTO BEANS

- Organic • BPA-free can • Sugar free

GRAINS

STEER CLEAR

RICE & BEANS

BETTY CROCKER CHICKEN HELPER CHICKEN FRIED RICE

It's a crock, all right! Phytate-loaded rice with partially hydrogenated soybean oil (GMO trans fat), irradiated spices (EMD), sugar (EMD), and numerous MSG ingredients. And how does this fried rice get its authentic fried appearance? That's easy. It is topped with caramel color (carcinogen) and four counterfeit colors!

BUSH'S BAKED BEANS

Your BPA-lined, canned, unsprouted beans are coated in brown and white sugar (EMD), irradiated spices, corn distilled GMO vinegar, modified cornstarch (GMO/MSG), and caramel colors (possible carcinogen).

VIGO SPANISH BEAN SOUP MIX

You will eat uncontrollably once you get this product's ten different forms of MSG into your belly! Your bowl also contains eight different GMO corn ingredients, three added forms of gluten, and three GMO soy products as well as GMO trans fats from partially hydrogenated corn, soy, and cottonseed oils. Imagine all that junk and you still have to cook it yourself!

☐ Choose organic rice and beans.

☐ Choose to ferment/sprout rice and beans.

☐ Choose white rice over brown rice.

☐ Choose BPA-free cans of beans or beans in bags.

☐ Avoid eating too much beans and rice—they're high in carbohydrates.

☐ Avoid eating more than two servings of rice per week to limit arsenic exposure.

☐ Avoid added Poor Food ingredients in your rice and bean mixes.

*My go-to Rich Food choices for rice and beans:*_____

Checkout Checklist

Aisle 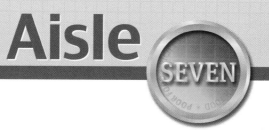 SEVEN

Baking

We are gathered here today not to say good-bye to your grandmother's secret recipe for Boston cream pie or your family's traditional tiramisu, nor do we want to put an end to your love affair with chocolate chip cookies and double chocolate brownies—we just want to improve the micronutrient quality of them. While it may be difficult at first to wrap your head around rewriting a family recipe to conform to our Rich Food, Poor Food philosophy, you will soon see that with just a few small changes in how you shop in the baking aisle, great-aunt Mary's scrumptious scones can easily become a healthy hybrid.

Sweeteners—La Dolce Vita (The Sweet Life)

IN CHAPTER 2, we reminded you about the hazards of sugar and introduced you to the Sinister Sugar Substitutes, so you may be asking yourself, *What do I use to sweeten my coffee or add to my homemade desserts?* Well, never fear—stevia is here.

Stevia

If you haven't yet heard of stevia, then you are in for a real treat because stevia is an all-natural sweetener that substitutes for sugar in almost any recipe. We actually grow stevia in our flower box and use the little green leaves in various dishes to add a touch of sweetness. You can pick up small seedlings at your local home improvement store's garden center.

However, don't be fooled by the different stevia products in most grocery stores—they are more like products that use stevia mixed with some kind of sugar base such as dextrose, maltodextrin, xylitol, or erythritol. While the xylitol or erythritol bases are better choices, we prefer pure stevia extract. The full name for stevia is *stevia rebaudiana*. If you see this as the only ingredient listed, you are looking at the real thing.

The stevia leaf contains compounds called steviol glycosides, which make it about thirty to forty-five times as sweet as sugar, but two of the glycosides—stevioside and rebaudioside—are approximately three hundred times as sweet as sugar. When most people taste stevia, they are surprised by how sweet it is. Stevia is fine for diabetics or even very low-carb dieters. In fact, some studies suggest that stevia can help reverse diabetes and metabolic syndrome and reduce hypertension.

Here is how it works. Rebaudiosides are metabolized into stevioside in the digestive tract, where it is broken down to glucose and steviol. The terrific benefit is *all* of the glucose is used by the bacteria in the colon and *not* absorbed into the bloodstream. Because steviol cannot be further digested, it is excreted by the body.

The stevia plant has been used in South America for more than fifteen hundred years and is widely chosen around the world as a safe, natural sweetener. It's our number one pick! Warning: if you are allergic to ragweed, stevia may not be for you, as it is a close relative and can sometimes cause similar allergic reactions.

Stevia's Sweet Siblings

Aside from stevia, you may (or may not) have heard about some other natural sweeteners, including agave nectar, xylitol, raw honey, and coconut sugar. While we like stevia over all these options, below is a small synopsis of each of these sweet siblings.

AGAVE NECTAR: It seems like agave nectar is in everything these days. While the name may conjure up natural goodness, this highly processed syrup contains more fructose than high fructose corn syrup—up to 80 percent more! While agave may be lower on the glycemic index, a study in the *Journal of Clinical Investigation* found that participants who consumed fructose gained more unhealthy visceral (belly) fat, were more insulin resistant, and were at greater risk for developing heart disease and diabetes than those consuming similar amounts of glucose. This is because fructose must go directly to the liver for processing, where it is more easily converted into fat that plain old glucose, which your body can burn immediately in the bloodstream. All in all, not a sweetener we recommend.

XYLITOL AND OTHER SUGAR ALCOHOLS: While this sweetener was originally made from birch bark, today's xylitol is a processed industrial product typically derived from wood or corn. Xylitol, along with erythritol, sorbitol, and mannitol, are sugar alcohols, which aren't absorbed by the body the way sugar is and therefore have a smaller effect on blood sugar. Because of this, they are often used in diabetic or low-carb food items. The term *net carbs* is often used when sugar alcohols are used in a product, meaning the total number of carbs minus any contributed by sugar alcohol. However, because nearly 80 percent of xylitol is metabolized through the liver, overuse could lead to damaging effects. Some people also report stomach upset and bloating after eating foods made with sugar alcohols. On the positive side, xylitol and all other sugar alcohols cannot be metabolized by oral bacteria and therefore do not contribute to tooth decay. Having said all this, we still like stevia better.

ORGANIC RAW HONEY: Did you know that raw honey is the only food that will never spoil? It's true. Our friend Diane Sanfilippo, author of *Practical Paleo,* made this her natural sweetener top pick. However, while organic raw honey is a much better choice than most sweeteners out there, it is still a form of sugar, so we recommend rare usage.

ORGANIC COCONUT SUGAR: This minimally processed cane sugar substitute comes packed with micronutrients and has a low glycemic score of only 35 (honey 55, sugar 61, agave nectar 30), which means it won't raise your blood sugar too high. It's a better option, but don't overdo it. While we still recommend stevia be used, this is another great option that works well in recipes.

• • • • • • • • • • • • • • • •

Flour

MUCH LIKE HOW WE SUGGESTED you swap your sugar for stevia, due to the adverse health consequences of eating wheat detailed earlier, it's time to give a facelift to your flour. Here's a tip: when rewriting your recipes, you need to replace flour by weight with a Rich Food replacement flour of similar texture. This isn't a cup-to-cup exchange, since your flour replacements may weigh in differently than conventional flour. Weigh the refined white flour required in a Poor Food recipe, and then match the weight with the replacement flour of your choice to make it a Rich Food recipe. Additionally, none of these flours work perfectly on their own. Combine their unique textures and flavors to find the perfect alternative flour combination for each recipe. Here are some alternative flours that we prefer and a few more tips for reworking your recipes.

Coconut Flour

This wheat alternative, made from the meat of the coconut, is fantastic to thicken sauces and to bake with. It is very low in carbohydrates and it contains lauric acid, which can help to increase your "good" cholesterol.

It adds a natural sweetness to any recipe. Tip: when adding coconut flour, you must add more liquid to the recipe because this flour readily absorbs moisture. Adding egg to the mixture will also help the coconut flour to act more like wheat flour. Coconut flour has no gluten, and the eggs take the place of gluten. Add four eggs for every half cup of coconut flour. It is best to use coconut flour in conjunction with another alternative flour, such as buckwheat or almond, in recipes.

Almond Flour (aka Almond Meal)

This alternative adds a nutty flavor to recipes and is fantastic in batters. Tip: it is best to use sprouted almond meal, which you can make yourself to save money. Simply follow directions to sprout them (see snacks, page 229), and then place them in a food processor until finely ground. That's all almond meal is, folks—ground almonds!

Buckwheat Flour

Don't be confused by the word *wheat* in *buckwheat*. This flour is not harvested from grain—buckwheat is a seed. It is a fantastic source of magnesium, very high in fiber, and one of the best sources of protein in the plant kingdom. It has a very strong, distinct flavor and creates darker, earthier dough. Tip: because buckwheat is a heavier flour, it is best exchanged for whole wheat flour in recipes.

Flax Meal

Flax meal is rich in omega-3 and adds a lot of fiber and a nutty flavor to any recipe. In baking, as a flour alternative, it can be too crumbly on its own. A better texture can be created when flax meal is used alongside almond meal or other nut meals. Two tablespoons of ground flaxseeds contains 2,400 mg of omega-3. While flax is not the best source of omega-3 because it does not contain EPA and DHA, it is great for vegetarians or vegans who may not consume enough omega-3s through the leading sources of fish or grass-fed meats. Tip: use a sprouted flax meal in lieu of the seeds in yogurt bowls and salads. The seeds are very small; if not chewed carefully, they may not get fully digested, and you would miss out on their omega-3 benefits. The sprouting not only reduces the phytic acid, but also increases enzyme and vitamin availability.

Chia Seeds

Ch-ch-ch-chia! Who would have thought that the "As Seen on TV" pet would harvest such incredible health benefits? These antioxidant-rich seeds supply a whopping 2,400 mg of vegetarian source omega-3 per tablespoon and offer a beneficial 3-to-1 ratio of anti-inflammatory omega-3 to inflammation-causing omega-6. Finely grinding chia seeds in a blender or food processor creates an alternative flour that works best when combined in recipes with our other alternative flour suggestions. Because chia can absorb more than twelve times its weight in water, it works as an excellent binder in gluten-free, wheat-free recipes. Try it as a replacement for breadcrumbs in meatballs and meatloaf as well. Tip: if substituting ground chia seed for flax meal, reduce by one-half to two-thirds. Always add chia to the wet mixture first and allow twenty minutes for it to absorb the liquid before adding it to the recipe.

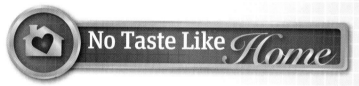

You didn't think we would tell you what kind of pancake syrup to use and leave you high and dry without a delicious, warm, fluffy pancake to enjoy it on, now did you?

Grain-Free and Guilt-Free Perfect Pancakes

INGREDIENTS

- ½ cup almond flour (sprouted if possible)
- ½ cup buckwheat flour (sprouted if possible)
- 1 tsp. baking powder

- 1 large pastured egg
- 1 tsp. pure vanilla extract
- 1 cup of organic milk or buttermilk (preferably unpasteurized, nonhomogenized)

- Pure stevia extract (or preferred sugar substitute) to taste
- 2 Tbsp. of melted grass-fed butter
- Grass-fed butter for greasing

DIRECTIONS

 1 Mix all of the dry ingredients together.

 2 In a separate bowl, mix together egg, sweetener, vanilla, milk, and melted butter.

 3 Slowly pour the wet ingredients into the dry ingredients while continually mixing so that no clumps form.

 4 Heat a frying pan or griddle, and grease with butter. Spoon batter into desired size of pancakes.

 5 Cook until small bubbles start to form, flip, and cook a bit longer.

 6 Serve with Triple Berry Syrup (page 171)

BAKING

Oil

ALMOST EVERY RECIPE CALLS FOR some kind of oil, so which is best? First, if you can substitute a high-quality, grass-fed butter for oil in a recipe, do it (melted, of course). This will enhance the flavor and give you all the benefits of conjugated linoleic acid (CLA) and the essential micronutrients found in grass-fed butter. If not, our next choice would be to use a cold pressed organic extra virgin coconut or palm oil. These oils are stable fats and are safe to use for high heat cooking or frying. When we refer to a type of fat as being stable, we mean that it is more saturated and hence less likely to suffer oxidate damage upon heating. Yep, saturated fat is good for you! After all, it's what our cell membranes are made out of, it's what many hormonal processes rely upon as a key raw material, and it's what our ancestors built those big brains on over the course of millions of years of human evolution. Most saturated fats are solid at room temperature and are not damaged by heat, air, and light as readily as unsaturated fats—such as monounsaturated (MUFAs) or polyunsaturated (PUFAs).

For you salad lovers out there, look for organic, cold pressed, extra virgin olive oil to go with your organic vinegar. Because of the high demand for olive oil, much of it is now being made with centrifuges and isn't "pressed" at all. True extra virgin comes exclusively from the first pressing of the olive paste, and the first pressing only. To make sure you are getting the best oil, look

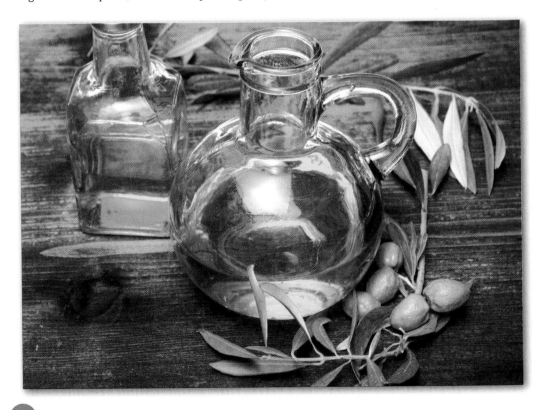

for the term *cold pressed* on the label. The European Union regulation states that the term *cold pressed* can only be used when the olive paste is kept at or below 27 degrees Celsius (80 degrees Fahrenheit) and when the oil is actually extracted with a press, not a centrifuge. Additionally, to ensure freshness, only buy oils from the current year's harvest. (Tip: if you subtract two years from the sell by date, you can usually determine when it was harvested.) The fresher the olive oil, the better. The International Olive Council has recently approved a method of measuring oil's polyphenol content—an indicator of its health-giving characteristics, taste, and shelf life. Ranging between 300 (low) to 800 (very high), an oil with a 500+ rating is optimal. They are not always listed, but the better products may have this number boasted on a label. Contact your brands of interest and inquire whether this olive oil is "first cold pressed extra virgin." Search for a domestic brand to ensure freshness, and stay away from the incredible bargains you see at big box stores of huge imported jugs of "extra virgin olive oil." Generally, imports are older and have less regulation of the use of the term *extra virgin* than domestic brands. Yes, you pay more for this Rich Food from domestic brands, but a truly fresh, pungent, sharp-tasting olive oil is one of the great indulgences of fine dining. A simple tip: if you detect a strong smell and taste, you've hit paydirt. If not, your extra-virgin choice is probably old and over-processed.

Last, take notice of what varietal of olive you enjoy in your olive oil. There are more than seven hundred kinds of olives in the world, and just like wines made from different grapes have vastly different flavor characteristics, you can make a hobby out of tasting a variety of olives to find your preferred oil. Using olive oil in your sauces and in low-heat simmered dishes is a terrific way to add depth and health to your dish. We don't recommend frying with olive oil; being monounsaturated, it is unstable at high heat and can easily oxidize.

Cold pressed nut and seed oils, such as peanut, sesame, avocado, macadamia, or flax work well in dressings and often hit an interesting nutty note. But don't cook with these oils—these fats oxidize when heated.

Two other great oils are fish oil (high in omega-3) and medium chain triglyceride (MCT) oil, which is derived from coconut oil and revs up the metabolism. You will probably have to go to a health food store or shop online to find these specialty options. While we don't use these oils for cooking, we do often use them on our salads and in our protein shakes.

Did you notice that we did not recommend corn, soybean, canola (rapeseed), safflower, cottonseed, or any vegetable oils at all? That is because these oils are heavily processed, often with high heat and chemical solvents. Before they go into those clear bottles that line the grocery store shelves (by the way, oil should be stored in dark bottles to protect from light), they are often chemically bleached, deodorized, and dyed yellow. Not to mention the fact that they are usually derived from GMO crops and are predominant in the pro-inflammatory omega-6 fatty acids that we are trying hard to minimize in favor of more anti-inflammatory omega-3s. Due to the adverse processing methods, you are essentially ingesting oxidized molecules that wreak immediate havoc on healthy cellular function. Yep, it's time to go back to butter! The bottom line is that these oils are not healthy and should be avoided at all costs.

And what about the canned cooking sprays? A quick inspection of their ingredient list is all it should take for you to recognize that most are made from the man-made oils we just gave the thumbs down to. Some even add in soy or wheat products as well as chemical anti-foaming agents. You may be surprised to learn how misleading the calories on the label can be. Read our review of the I Can't Believe It's Not Butter spray on page 83 for an eye-opening perspective. If you need to grease a pan or baking dish, just slather a stick of Rich Food butter or coconut oil on the surface. It's simple and fun, and you protect yourself from free radical damage.

If you need to spray oil, you can purchase an inexpensive oil spritzer from a specialty kitchen supply company and fill it with a Rich Food oil option. You can check out our favorite spritzers in the Rich Food Resource Center at CaltonNutrition.com.

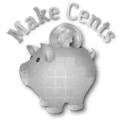

Don't spend more money than you need to on oils. Use the fat from your grass-fed beef or pastured pork (bacon), chicken, or duck to cook other components of your meal. We love our vegetables cooked under our chicken in the rotisserie, and our eggs cooked in that morning's bacon grease. You can collect and store these drippings in a canning jar right on your kitchen counter. This natural fat is not only healthy and temperature stable, it's free and tastes great.

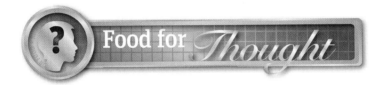

Food for Thought

Gotta get some ghee (pronounced with a hard G)! Ghee, the traditional clarified butter used in India, is a great substitute for oils. Made by heating butter to remove the milk proteins (casein), sugars, and water, ghee is extremely stable and doesn't require refrigeration. You can find ghee flavored with organic spices at specialty stores or make your own. Look for an organic, nonhomogenized grass-fed ghee to ensure that only the highest quality milk with the greatest micronutrient benefits has been used. Beware: ghee imported from India may contain *unlabeled* BHT. The Indian government allows for up to 2 percent of the total content to consist of those banned preservatives without labeling.

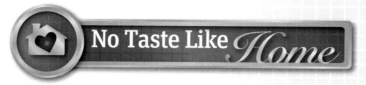

No Taste Like *Home*

Once you have located a source for local grass-fed, unpasteurized butter,
we suggest you make a batch of ghee. It doesn't require refrigeration,
which makes it perfect to pack for picnics and travel.

Ghee-licious Clarified Butter

INGREDIENT So simple, you need just one!

- The best Rich Food unsalted butter you can find. Preferably an organic, local, grass-fed, unpasteurized butter.

DIRECTIONS

 1 Place butter in a saucepan over low to moderate heat and melt. Do not cover.

 2 Bring butter to a simmer (light boil). You will notice milk solids foaming on top.

 3 Remove the froth with a clean spoon and continue simmering.

 4 Ghee is completed when the second foam appears on the surface and the liquid beneath turns golden and clear.

 5 Pour contents of saucepan through a strainer lined with cheesecloth to remove brown solids formed at the bottom. Store in an opaque, airtight canning jar.

 6 No need to refrigerate ghee.

GARLIC-INFUSED GHEE: *Add six garlic cloves for every four ounces of butter to the saucepan at the beginning of simmering. Strain ghee through cheesecloth-lined strainer. Cloves captured in cheesecloth can be used for other dishes at a later time.*

BAKING

Vinegar

VINEGAR HAS BEEN USED as a health tonic since the time of Hippocrates (460–377 BC), who prescribed it for curing persistent coughs. Consisting mainly of water and acetic acid, vinegar is produced through the fermentation of alcohol by acetic acid bacteria. Today we use vinegar in the kitchen, but in the past it was used as a mild acid for a wide variety of industrial, medical, and domestic uses. There are many distinct types and flavors of vinegar, including apple cider, balsamic, beer, cane, coconut, date, distilled, East Asian black, flavored, fruit, honey, Job's tears, kiwifruit, kombucha, malt, palm, raisin, rice, sinamak, spirit, sherry, white, and wine.

Some of the world's finest balsamic vinegar is aged for more than one hundred years. When choosing vinegar, it's fun to experiment. We like hot pepper infused vinegars to add a little kick to salad or a main dish. Just make sure when you are buying vinegar to get a quality organic product. This is because some vinegar is made from corn (GMO alert) and others from apples or grapes, which are both found at the top of the Terrible Twenty list. Additionally, some brands of balsamic vinegar are just mixtures of concentrated grape juice and vinegar, laced with caramel and sugar—definitely a Steer Clear. Remember to look for amber or opaque bottles to protect your vinegar's nutrients, flavor, and color from the damaging effects of light.

• • • • • • • • • • • • • • •

Soy Sauce

FROM SUSHI TO STIR-FRIES, this Asian ingredient is a must-have for the pantry. The name alone reveals its potential for GMOs. However, you might not be aware what other Poor Food hazards are also lurking in soy sauce. This salty sauce is almost always made with wheat and MSG, so read labels carefully to avoid these unwanted ingredients. Your best two options are either to opt for an organic soy-based product, or, if like us, you have opted to keep wheat and soy out of your diet (see soy reasoning under soy milk on 56), try coconut aminos instead. You may be surprised to find out that coconut aminos, created from the sap of a coconut tree, taste almost exactly like soy sauce. This soy sauce substitute is high in protein building blocks called amino acids that can enhance overall brain activity, boost immune system, and increase physical energy levels.

• • • • • • • • • • • • • • •

Cocoa

LOVE CHOCOLATE, BUT DON'T EAT IT anymore because you are staying away from added sugar? Well, let's end your misery right now: 100 percent natural organic cocoa doesn't contain any added sugar, and it can be combined with a little stevia to enjoy the wonderful taste of chocolate. The antioxidant level of dark chocolate rivals or exceeds even some of the most potent fruits and vegetables, making it a Rich Food in every sense of the word. Like vinegar, chocolate has a long history. Evidence of cacao beverages date back to 1,900 BC. And although its best to enjoy cocoa in moderation due to its oxalic acid content (one of the only negatives about cocoa; there had to be something, right?), some research has suggested that dark chocolate can help prevent heart disease and lower blood pressure. Other research has shown chocolate to boost cognitive abilities and lower cholesterol levels. Melting chocolate in one's mouth produced an increase in brain activity and heart rate more intense than those associated with passionate kissing, and the effect lasted four times longer! Now that is *hot* chocolate. If you are a chocolate lover, you can look forward to our No Taste Like Home chocolate bark recipe in Aisle 8: Snacks.

STEER HERE

STEVIA

KAL PURE STEVIA EXTRACT

- Pure stevia extract
- Doesn't spike insulin
- Best powdered formula for use in hot beverages
- KAL also makes an organic version, but it has a more metallic, less preferred flavor

STEVITA SIMPLY STEVIA POWDER/ DROPS AND FLAVORED DROPS

- Pure stevia extract
- Doesn't spike insulin
- Multiple flavored drops available

SWEETLEAF ORGANIC STEVIA EXTRACT POWDER AND SWEET DROPS

- Pure stevia extract
- Doesn't spike insulin
- Multiple flavored drops available

SWEET SIBLINGS

SWEETTREE ORGANIC COCONUT SUGAR + STEVIA BY BIG TREE FARMS

- Organic stevia and palm sugar
- Very low glycemic index

COCONUT SECRET'S COCONUT NECTAR OR CRYSTALS

- Organic
- Low glycemic index

ORGANIC BEE FARMS 100% RAW HONEY

- Organic
- Raw
- Rich in micronutrients

FLOUR

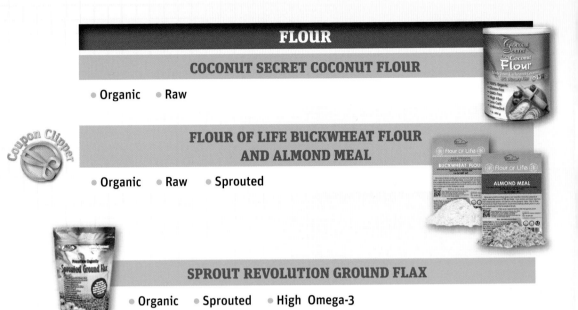

COCONUT SECRET COCONUT FLOUR

- Organic
- Raw

FLOUR OF LIFE BUCKWHEAT FLOUR AND ALMOND MEAL

Coupon Clipper

- Organic
- Raw
- Sprouted

SPROUT REVOLUTION GROUND FLAX

- Organic
- Sprouted
- High Omega-3

OIL

Coupon Clipper

KASANDRINOS EXTRA VIRGIN OLIVE OIL

- Organic
- Cold pressed
- Opaque container

DR. BRONNER'S MAGIC ALL ONE COCONUT OIL

- Organic
- Fresh pressed virgin
- Fair trade

Try the whole kernel.

NUTIVA ORGANIC EXTRA VIRGIN COCONUT OIL

- Organic
- Cold pressed

SPECTRUM SHORTENING

- Organic
- Expeller Pressed Palm oil shortening is great for baking crusts and crisping fries

SPECTRUM ARBEQUINA EXTRA VIRGIN OLIVE OIL

- Organic
- Cold pressed
- Unfiltered
- Opaque container

GHEE

PURE INDIAN 100% ORGANIC GRASS-FED GHEE

- Organic
- From grass-fed, non-homogenized butter
- Available in six different flavor varieties

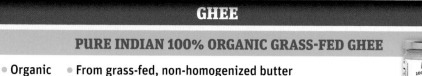

VINEGAR

EDEN APPLE CIDER VINEGAR

- Organic
- Raw
- Unpasteurized
- Opaque container

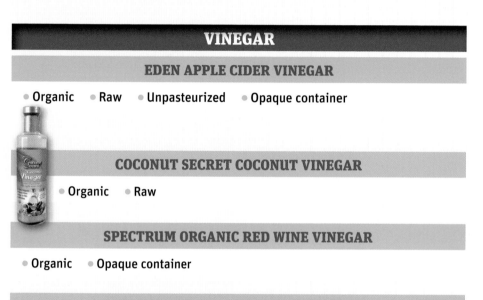

COCONUT SECRET COCONUT VINEGAR

- Organic
- Raw

SPECTRUM ORGANIC RED WINE VINEGAR

- Organic
- Opaque container

COLAVITA ORGANIC BALSAMIC VINEGAR

- Organic
- Opaque container

SOY SAUCE

SAN-J ORGANIC GLUTEN-FREE TAMARI SOY SAUCE PLATINUM

- Organic
- Gluten-free

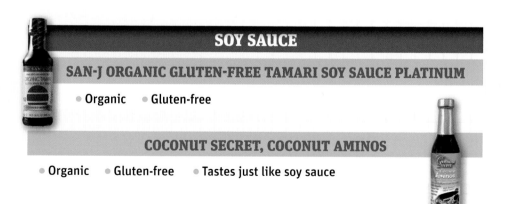

COCONUT SECRET, COCONUT AMINOS

- Organic
- Gluten-free
- Tastes just like soy sauce

CACAO

DAGOBA ORGANIC UNSWEETENED CHOCOLATE FOR BAKING

- Organic

Also try their cocoa powder.

BAKER'S UNSWEETENED CHOCOLATE

- The best sugar-free grocery store option for baking

HERSHEY'S COCOA SPECIAL DARK 100% CACAO

- The best sugar-free grocery store option for powdered chocolate

STEER CLEAR

TRUVIA

Truvia uses a patent-pending form of stevia called Rebiana, created by the health-conscious folks at Coca-Cola and Cargill, who reportedly derive Rebiana from stevia leaves through a forty-two-step process that uses chemicals, including acetone, methanol, acetonitrile, isopropanol, tert-butanol, and "mixtures thereof." Rebiana is also combined with the sugar alcohol erythritol. While erythritol is considered a zero-calorie sweetener in the United States, the European Union currently labels it (and all other sugar alcohols) as containing 2.4 calories per gram. Stick to pure stevia extract.

TRUVIA BAKING BLEND WITH SUGAR

As if Rebiana and erythritol weren't bad enough, on top of it all, the baking blend adds sugar in! We thought we were trying to find a sugar substitute to get this everyday micronutrient depleter (EMD) out of our diets. Truvia is truly confused.

STEVIA IN THE RAW AND BAKER'S BAG

Mixes stevia with dextrose and maltodextrin; both sugars are derived from corn (GMO).

ALL WHITE REFINED FLOUR, BAKING FLOUR, ALL-PURPOSE FLOUR, WHOLE WHEAT FLOURS

Gluten wheat belly alert!

ALLEGRO VINTAGE BALSAMIC VINEGAR MARINADE

A perfect example of what you do not want. First, the balsamic vinegar used in this product is made from high fructose corn syrup (GMO, EMD) and then is combined with brown sugar (EMD), soy sauce (made from hydrolyzed soy protein (GMO, MSG), corn syrup (GMO), and caramel coloring (possible carcinogen). Stick to the real stuff.

HOUSE OF TSANG SOY SAUCE

GMO-likely soybeans combined with four forms of MSG (hydrolyzed soy and wheat proteins along with disodium ionsinate and disodium guanylate) and sodium benzoate (possible carcinogen). The only ingredient in this soy sauce that we don't dislike is water.

SHUFRA BITTERSWEET BAKING BARS

Don't be fooled by baking bar imposters like this one, which are unhealthy concoctions of sugar, cocoa, hydrogenated vegetable oils, and artificial flavor.

GREAT VALUE MILK CHOCOLATE FLAVORED HOT COCOA MIX WITH MARSHMALLOWS MADE WITH REAL COCOA

Not the same as the 100 percent cocoas above, this *made with* real cocoa product's first three ingredients are sugar (EMD), whey (MSG), and corn syrup solids (EMD, GMO) joined by more sugar (EMD), corn syrup (EMD, GMO), modified cornstarch (GMO), gelatin (MSG), artificial flavor, partially hydrogenated soybean oil (trans fats), mono and diglycerides (trans fats), and more artificial flavor.

BAKING

❑ Choose pure stevia extract to sweeten.

❑ Choose coconut sugar, raw honey, or sugar alcohols as secondary substitutes for sugar.

❑ Choose alternate flours such as coconut flour, almond flour, buckwheat flour, and flax meal.

❑ Choose coconut oil or palm oil for high-temperature heating and frying.

❑ Choose grass-fed organic butter as replacement for oil when possible.

❑ Choose cold pressed, extra virgin olive oil or cold pressed nut and seed oils for salads and sauces.

❑ Choose only organic, gluten-free soy sauce or coconut aminos.

❑ Choose organic vinegar with low sugar content.

❑ Choose organic unsweetened cocoa.

❑ Avoid throwing away the fat after cooking quality meats. Retain it for later use.

❑ Avoid grain-based flours.

❑ Avoid clear glass containers for oil and vinegar.

❑ Avoid all man-made, highly processed vegetable oils, including corn, soybean, canola (rapeseed), safflower, and cottonseed.

My go-to Rich Food choices for baking: _____

_____

_____

_____

_____

_____

_____

_____

A Rack of Riches

These herbs and spices add great flavors to your foods and have some incredible health benefits. Experimenting with a variety of spices and flavors can assist you in serving up a full spectrum of health benefits.

CAUTION: most grocery store spices are irradiated. Remember, irradiation, an EMD we introduced you to in Chapter 2, is the process of exposing food to radiation in order to destroy microorganisms, bacteria, viruses, or insects that might be present in the food. While irradiation works to kill bacteria, it also disrupts the structure of everything it passes through. Specifically, irradiation breaks up a food's DNA, vitamins, minerals, and proteins and creates free radicals (atoms, molecules, or ions that contain unpaired electrons and crash into each other, multiplying exponentially), which contribute to many degenerative diseases, including heart disease, dementia, cancer, and cataracts.

Additionally, irradiation destroys the essential micronutrients that can help you reach micronutrient sufficiency. Your spice rack has so much to offer—that is, when you buy the Rich Food option, which is always the non-irradiated organic spice—our top pick.

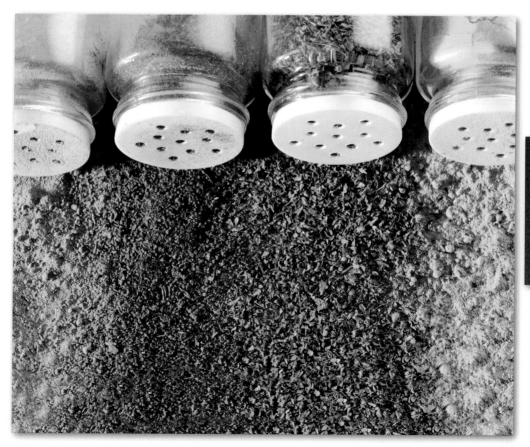

BAKING

The Spice Superhighway

Dill

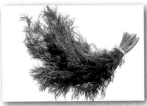

HELPS YOUR DIGESTION. A teaspoon a day can reduce 80 percent of bloating in only three days. Its antibacterial oils not only kill any possible stomach bugs but also help in the breakdown of carbohydrates and proteins.

USES: Feathery texture is sharp tasting. Great on fish, in chicken, and in potato salads. Used in pickling.

Tarragon

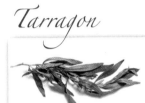

FOR HEART HEALTH. One teaspoon daily can lower LDL cholesterol more than 40 percent while increasing good cholesterol nearly 30 percent. Tarragon contains a chemical called rutin, which boosts circulation and reduces plaque in the arteries.

USES: Flavor of anise, licorice, mint, hay, and pine. Try it in Bernaise sauce.

Oregano

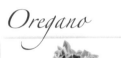

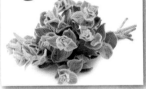

BACTERIA BE GONE. Due to the high levels of antibacterial compounds and antioxidants, oregano is just as effective at killing E. coli and staph bacteria as penicillin.

USES: Tastes robust. Best in tomato dishes, usually of Mediterranean or Mexican origin.

Bay Leaf

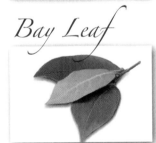

NATURAL PAIN RELIEVER. Eliminates headaches and migraines. Bay leaf is rich in eugenol, a natural anesthetic that alleviates pain.

USES: Tastes woody. Perfect in soups, sauces, stews, and pot roasts.

Sage

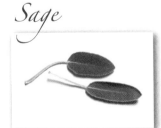

MEMORY MINDER. Both the phytonutrients and volatile oils in sage maintain levels of acetylcholine, a neurotransmitter that supports memory.

USES: Piney with eucalyptus notes. Lovely addition to stuffing and pork dishes.

Cayenne

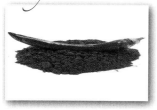

APPETITE SUPPRESSANT AND METABOLISM BOOSTER. Capsaicin, found in cayenne, has thermogentic properties that increase your blood flow and metabolism. Individuals who only use cayenne infrequently also find it reduces hunger.

USES: Sweet heat. Works well with meats and cheeses.

Cinnamon

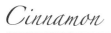

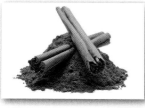

CONTROLS GLUCOSE LEVELS. Cinnamon contains antioxidants called polyphenols that boost levels of three key proteins responsible for insulin signaling, glucose transport, and inflammatory response. Sprinkle half a teaspoon on your food to slow carbohydrate absorption by 29 percent.

USES: Sweet and savory. This spice is found in almost all world cuisine. From stews to pies, this spice doesn't discriminate.

Cardamom

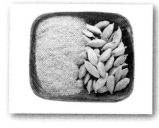

TREATS INDIGESTION. Chew one teaspoon of these seeds to soothe a sour belly. The aroma and therapeutic properties of cardamom are due to the volatile oil in its seed, which contains cineol, terpinene, limonene, sabinene, and terpineol.

USES: Pungent and sweet. This fragrant spice is used in rich curries and milk-based preparations as well as in spice cakes and desserts.

Rosemary

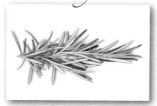

THE BRAIN BOOSTER AND FATIGUE FIGHTER. With just one sniff, the phytochemicals found in rosemary can rev up your mind by increasing the production of beta waves. Carnosol, a nutrient unique to this herb, fights fatigue by flushing out energy-sapping toxins from the body.

USES: Smell rosemary sprigs to increase alertness in only five minutes. Intense pine flavor. Great on grilled meats and adds an interesting boost to chocolate desserts.

AND OUR FAVORITE RICH FOOD SPICE IS . . . TURMERIC

This mildly woody spice is a key ingredient in many Indian, Persian, and Thai dishes. This "poor man's" saffron is rich in benefits. The active ingredient, curcumin, is so powerful that it is commonly made into expensive nutraceutical capsules.

According to Ajay Goel, PhD, Director of Epigenetics and Cancer Prevention at Baylor Research Institute in Dallas, "Curcumin is a complete well-being tonic—it benefits every organ in the body . . . It shows promise of fighting nearly every disease."

Dr. Goel suggests that curcumin aids in the prevention of Alzheimer's, Parkinson's, cancer, heart disease, diabetes, arthritis, and depression.

Why not just cook up a cure in your kitchen tonight?

CURCUMIN CONTROLS BLOOD SUGAR: It switches on the liver genes that keep glucose levels in check. It improves the pancreas's ability to make insulin and helps slow down the metabolism of carbohydrates after meals.

CURCUMIN FIGHTS CANCER: It inhibits the genetic switches that allow for cancerous cell growth to occur.

CURCUMIN SPEEDS UP METABOLISM: USDA research shows that is enhances cellular energy to speed metabolism.

CURCUMIN CLEARS PLAQUE: It removes amyloyd plaque buildup in the brain that can cause Alzheimer's.

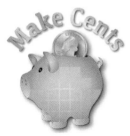

Let's face it, the organic spice jars in this aisle are small and pricey, and it can take a long time to use up some of these specialty ingredients. Your best bet is to buy your organic spices in the bulk section of your local health food or specialty spice store, where you can buy smaller amounts of the spices you need right away. This guarantees that your spices are fresh and loaded with flavor, and it saves you money when a recipe only calls for a pinch. Buy your own glass jars online or wash out old spice jars and transfer contents from store baggies into convenient glass jars. Store them in a cool, dark place to prevent oxidative damage from light and oxygen.

Viva Vanilla!

WHEN CHOOSING VANILLA for your favorite recipe, purchase pure vanilla extract and leave behind the less expensive imitation vanilla. Here's why. Most imitation vanilla is actually vanillan, a singular flavor created either as a by-product from the pulp used in making commercial paper products or derived from coal tar—both unnatural processes. Real vanilla beans have 171 identified aromatic taste components, far more complex and intensely flavored than the imitation vanilla. You need twice as much imitation vanilla in a recipe as the real thing to obtain a similar essence. So while pure vanilla extract may cost a little more, you can buy less and get the real deal.

Also, the word *pure* on labels can be a misleading misfit. Many expensive brands add sugar into the mix. Once sugar is added, the vanilla is no longer pure (at least by our standards), but it can still be labeled as such. Read labels!

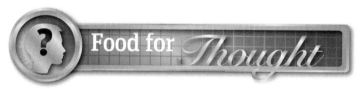

Steer clear of expensive spice mixes and premade rubs. Most of these products add in sugar, dextrose, evaporated cane juice, and other sweeteners. Additionally, many add in wheat, and the added salt is most likely refined (see the next section for more on the salt refinement process). Take a detour around these high sugar and sodium products and mix your own. Get shakin' on your creativity, and then store your favorite mixed combinations in clean glass jars on your spice rack.

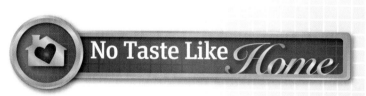

Ragin' Cajun Blackening Blend

Looking to spice up your meats or seafood? Make a batch of this blend and keep it handy for nights when you are looking to add a little kick in your kitchen. Store in an airtight container.

INGREDIENTS

- 1 Tsp. organic garlic powder
- 2 Tbsp. organic paprika
- 1 Tbsp. organic ground dried thyme
- 1 Tbsp. organic ground dried oregano

- 1 Tbsp. organic cayenne pepper (dare you to add double!)
- 1 tsp. organic ground black pepper
- 1 tsp. organic ground white pepper

A Sea of Salts

WHILE SALT IS A STAPLE in every kitchen and restaurant, what do we really know about it? As it turns out, salt has a long and colorful history. For example, *salary* comes from the Latin word *sal* (salt) because Romans were often paid in salt. Around 110 BC, salt was considered so valuable that salt piracy was punishable by death! During the Age of Discovery (the fifteenth to seventeenth centuries), Africans and European explorers valued salt ounce for ounce on par with gold.

Okay, so salt has an interesting history—but salt is salt, right? Well, no. There are a handful of salts that we are all familiar with, like table salt, kosher salt, sea salt, and even "no-salt" salt alternatives, but would you be surprised to know that none of these salts are natural salts? That's right—none of these salts, including even our beloved sea salt, exists in nature. All of these salts have been refined (processed).

Similar to wheat and sugar, which have been processed to make refined white flour and refined white sugar, almost all of the salt consumed in the United States has been processed to make refined white salt. This refined salt is added to nearly all grocery store goodies and restaurant recipes—at the expense of your health.

So, what's the difference between refined and unrefined salt? In its unrefined natural state, salt is not bright white but slightly gray, brownish, or pink. Unrefined salt is also jam-packed with more than ninety minerals, including sodium, chloride, calcium, magnesium, potassium, iodine, silicon, sulfur, phosphorus, and vanadium. During the refining process—the sole purpose of which is to create a better-preserved, more appealing dry white salt—all of the salt's essential minerals, except sodium and chloride, are stripped away and replaced with toxic chemical anti-caking agents that work to prevent the salt from mixing with water and clumping, both in the salt package (good) and in your body (not good).

While iodine has been added back into many salts, thus marketed as "iodized," it is only one of more than ninety minerals that had been removed. In addition, in some cases, dextrose (a form of sugar made from GMO corn) has also been introduced. Would you ever have expected sugar to be hiding in your salt? In its unrefined state, salt is health promoting—in fact, it is essential for life. Unrefined salt still contains minerals and electrolytes that enable your body to utilize the sodium and chloride properly.

But make sure to read the labels carefully. As stated earlier, these product billboards are often misleading. While your sea salt may say it is "natural," check the fine print to find out if it has been refined. If there is no fine print, the rule of thumb is: if the salt is white in color, it has been refined! You can help fight fatigue, adrenal disorders, headaches, thyroid disorders, and lower cholesterol levels and high blood pressure just by sprinkling on the smart salt—an unrefined one, steeped in its salty goodness.

Become Passionate About Pepper

WHILE WATER AND SALT ARE THE FIRST AND SECOND most added ingredients in recipes around the globe, pepper (ground peppercorns) is third. Pepper is the oldest and most widely used spice, accounting for a full one-fourth of the world's spice trade. First cultivated as long ago as 1,000 BC, the pungent flavor of the peppercorn was prized for its flavor-enhancing abilities and medicinal properties (digestive stimulant, expectorant, skin afflictions, and hives).

While there are seemingly many varieties of peppercorns, they all really come from the same vine, *Piper nigrum*. Peppercorns are picked and prepared at different times in the ripening process and in different ways to achieve their unique white, black, green, and red colors. True red pepper is extremely rare, and most references to it are actually referring to rosé, or pink pepper, which isn't really a pepper at all, but rather a dried berry found only on the island of Réunion in the Indian Ocean.

As with all spices, it is imperative to purchase organic pepper if you want to avoid irradiation and other potentially harmful pesticide residue. Pepper has been found to have antioxidant properties and anti-carcinogenic effects. Additionally, piperine, a substance present in black pepper, acts as a thermogenic compound, increases happiness-inducing serotonin and beta-endorphin production in the brain, and dramatically increases absorption of selenium, B vitamins, beta-carotene, curcumin, and other micronutrients.

Variety	Taste	Use
Green Peppercorn	Clean and crisp and not complex in flavor	Perfect for fish
White Peppercorn	Clean, clear heat	Preferred in Thai and Indian recipes
Tellicherry Black Peppercorn	Complex and overflowing with flavor	A fine black pepper choice to add interest to meatier dishes
Rose Peppercorn	Mild and slightly acidic with a hint of sweetness	Perfect for nouveau cuisine

BAKING

STEER HERE

SPICES

SIMPLY ORGANIC BRAND SPICES

Offers a fantastic variety of organic spices.

FRONTIER ORGANIC SPICES

Offers a fantastic variety of organic spices.

SMITH AND TRUSLOW ORGANIC SPICES

- Dated, smaller opaque jars keep the spices fresher longer

MORTON & BASSETT ORGANIC SPICES

They also have a line of non-organic, non-irradiated spices on store shelves.

VANILLA

SIMPLY ORGANIC MADAGASCAR PURE VANILLA EXTRACT

- No sugar added

SALT & PEPPER

REAL SALT

- Unrefined with full spectrum mineral content.

Other great salts to consider are Celtic, Himalayan, lava sea salt, Fleur de Sel, and French grey.

EPICUREAN ORGANICS PEPPERCORNS

Offers a fantastic variety of organic peppercorns.

MCCORMICK GOURMET COLLECTION 100% ORGANIC GROUND PEPPER

- Organic   - Available in many grocery stores

SPICES

SPICE ISLAND, MCCORMICK SPICES

These irradiated, non-organic spices are free-radical fallouts.

VANILLA

NIELSON-MASSEY PURE VANILLA EXTRACTS

Fancy cooking equipment outlets like Williams Sonoma and Sur La Table should know better than to sell vanilla that contains sugar.

SALT & PEPPER

MORTON SALT

This table salt, and other refined white table salts like it, contains dextrose (GMO corn).

KOSHER SALT

Don't let the coarse texture fool you—it is still refined!

IRRADIATED BLACK PEPPER

Any time it is not organic, you need to run from the free radicals. Time to pick an organic pepper.

BAKING

☐ **Choose organic spices.**

☐ **Choose pure (not imitation) vanilla extract with no sugar added.**

☐ **Choose unrefined sea salt.**

☐ **Choose organic pepper.**

☐ Avoid irradiated spices.

☐ Avoid added sugar.

☐ Avoid white table salt.

*My go-to Rich Food choices for spices:*_____

_____

_____

_____

_____

_____

_____

_____

_____

_____

_____

_____

_____

_____

_____

_____

Aisle

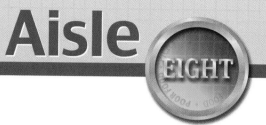

EIGHT

• •

Snacks

cience has discovered that your seemingly uncontrollable cravings are not caused by a natural desire for potato chips or ice cream, but rather by a deficiency of certain essential micronutrients. In *Naked Calories,* we explained that cravings for salty foods are often caused by calcium deficiencies, while cravings for sweets can often be blamed on magnesium and calcium deficiencies. Luckily, you've been building your micronutrient sufficiency aisle by aisle, so there is less chance that these cravings will take hold. But even the most well-intentioned, disciplined, nutrition-conscious person is still human, craving a nibble of something sweet or salty now and then.

When these times of vulnerability strike, the secret to avoiding self-sabotage is to properly prepare. This means stocking your pantry with healthy Rich Food options for when these snack attacks sneak up. No, we aren't going to let you off the hook and tell you to buy 100-calorie snack packs or low-fat ice cream. In this aisle, as with all the others, we must examine the ingredients carefully. After all, they call it junk food for a reason.

Nuts and Seeds

DIFFICULT TO STOP EATING after just one taste, nuts are plentiful in a jar, but in nature, you would have had to work overtime to collect them. Our ancestors painstakingly gathered nuts and had to crack them open manually, one at a time. A single handful was quite a bounty! Not so today, as modern food manufacturers deliver them by the jarful, already shelled for your convenience. It's best to temper your taste buds and enjoy them for the time-consuming treasures that they really are.

Not only are nuts calorie-dense, which is why nature packaged them individually, but they invariably contain more pro-inflammatory omega-6s than omega-3s. However, nuts and seeds are loaded with micronutrients, too, so by all means, enjoy these Rich Foods, but eat them responsibly.

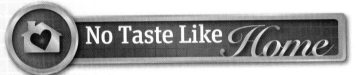

Nuts and seeds naturally contain the Everyday Micronutrient Depleter phytic acid. Sprouting and soaking nuts and seeds can be beneficial in reducing the phytic acid content while deactivating protease inhibitors meant to protect nuts and seeds from insects. This is great news because these same protease inhibitors can also prevent protease enzymes from digesting protein in the human digestive tract. Undigested proteins burden the pancreas and are thought to contribute to increased risk of pancreatic cancer. Soaking makes nuts and seeds significantly more nutritious, so it is best to purchase them sprouted or follow these simple steps.

Simply Soaked Nuts and Seeds

DIRECTIONS

 1 Place your choice of nuts or seeds in a bowl with enough filtered water to cover completely. Add salt into the water. See the noted amount for your nut/seed choice in the chart, opposite page.

 3 When time is up, rinse thoroughly. You can dry nuts and/or seeds in a dehydrator or on a cookie sheet in the oven on low heat with the door open. Don't overcook.

 2 Soak for the time listed in the chart below. You should drain and refill the water three to four times during the allotted soaking time.

 4 Store in an airtight container in the refrigerator.

KNOW YOUR NUTS, STUDY YOUR SEEDS

Nut/Seed	Soaking time Salt needed per 4 cups nuts or seeds	Protein*	Carbohy-drates*	Fat*	Omega-3*	Omega-6*	Calories
ALMOND (pasteurized almonds will not sprout)	Soak: 12 hrs. Salt: 1 tbsp.	6.0	6.1	14.0	.002	3.4	163
BRAZIL	Soak: none Salt: N/A	4.1	3.5	18.8	.005	5.8	186
CASHEW	Soak: 2 hrs. Salt: 1 tbsp.	5.2	8.6	12.4	.002	2.2	157
PEANUT	Soak: 8 hrs. Salt: 1 tbsp.	7	4.5	14.0	0	4.4	159
HAZELNUT	Soak: 8 hrs. Salt: 1 tbsp.	4.2	4.7	17.2	.02	2.2	178
MACADAMIA	Soak: none Salt: N/A	2.2	3.9	21.5	.06	0.4	204
PECAN	Soak: 8 hrs. Salt: 2 tsp.	2.6	3.9	20.4	0.3	5.8	196
PISTACHIO	Soak: none Salt: N/A	5.8	7.8	12.9	.07	3.7	159
WALNUT	Soak: 4 hrs. Salt: 2 tsp.	4.3	3.9	18.5	2.5	10.7	185
PINE	Soak: none Salt: N/A	3.8	3.7	19.4	.03	9.4	188
PUMPKIN	Soak: 6 hrs. Salt: 2 tbsp.	9.3	5.0	13.9	.05	5.8	151
FLAX	Soak: 8 hrs. Salt: 1 tsp.	1.8	8.1	9.3	5.3	1.7	149
CHIA	Soak: 2 hrs. Salt: 1 tsp.	5.8	11.6	9.3	5.5	1.6	140
SESAME	Soak: 8 hrs. Salt: 2 tsp.	5.0	6.6	8.6	0.1	6.0	160
SUNFLOWER	Soak: 2 hrs. Salt: 2 tbsp.	5.5	5.6	14.1	.02	6.5	164

* grams per one-ounce serving

SNACKS

Snacks That Go Crunch

WHILE ONLY A FEW YEARS AGO we may have had to sacrifice this snack choice, manufacturers now supply us with a few creative offerings we can really get behind. Our top picks for salty, crunchy treats utilize healthy vegetables, grains, seeds, and tubers (potatoes) as their bases. For example, while most corn in this country is GMO, you may be surprised to learn that popcorn is not made from GMO corn. This is great news in the snack aisle. The bad news, however, is that most bagged pre-popped popcorn is usually popped in man-made, inexpensive GMO oils. It's the oil used for popping and frying these snacks that really helps us de-

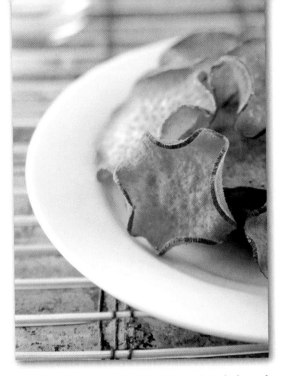

termine which chip to chuck. Another concern is that some common chip bases, such as kale and potatoes, are on the Terrible Twenty. Hence, you should choose organic brands to avoid pesticides.

Alternate Route to *Health*

Snacks made from sea vegetables make an excellent alternative to traditional chips, but you'll have to step out of the snack aisle to find them. Due to the versatility of sea vegetables like kelp and dulse, grocers haven't yet determined a permanent aisle for them. Your best bet for now is to ask a store employee to direct you.

Sea vegetable snacks can be eaten right out of their bags or crisped in an oven for a more chip-like texture. They also supply some extra benefits because sea vegetables are rich in iodine, a mineral often deficient in Westernized diets. Iodine controls the functioning of the thyroid gland in the human body, which in turn has a significant influence on the metabolic processes in the body. So you may see your metabolism rev up your energy levels and metabolic function regulate in part due to eating some sea vegetable snacks.

Say bye-bye to the bags and hello to homemade. Create your own veggie chips that are healthy and downright delicious, too!

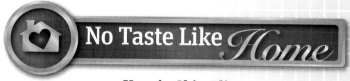
No Taste Like *Home*

Veggie Chip Flip

We like to make this recipe using organic sweet potatoes, carrots, organic zucchini, and organic kale and toss them together in a bowl for a great party mix. Your vegetable of choice can also be used, but remember to purchase organic if your veggie of choice is on the Terrible Twenty.

INGREDIENTS

- Organic extra virgin coconut oil at room temperature (enough to coat but not soak your vegetables)
- Unrefined sea salt
- Veggies of choice

DIRECTIONS

 1 Preheat oven to 375 degrees (350 degrees for kale chips)

 2 Wash vegetables (use the produce wash recipe on page 143)

3 Cut vegetables to desired shape and thickness

- Slice carrots thin on a mandolin, or for a dramatic, long chip, use a Y-shaped peeler and slice carrots by hand lengthwise.
- Zucchini and sweet potatoes are best cut round and thin.
- Always remove the stem when preparing kale chips, and cut or tear the leaves into bite-size chips. Remember, they will shrink when cooked, so make the pieces larger than your bite so you are not left with teeny scraps after baking.

 4 Coat the vegetable slices in oil, and sprinkle with organic salt and spices if desired.

 5 Coat a baking sheet with a thin layer of coconut oil.

6 Arrange the vegetables on the tray so that they do not overlap. The edges can touch, but only one type of vegetable should be on each tray.

 7 Bake for the time listed, or until the edges appear to be getting brown and crispy while the middles are still soft. Time varies greatly depending on how thin you prepared the slices. For thicker vegetable slices, you may want to flip halfway through cooking time.

Carrots: 10 to 15 minutes

Zucchini: Up to 30 minutes depending on water content and thickness

Sweet potatoes: 15 to 20 minutes

Kale: 8 to 10 minutes

 8 Remove from oven, and allow five minutes for firming before serving.

OPTION 1: Spice them up! If the bagged chips can do it, so can you. Use our Ragin' Cajun seasoning mix on page 221.

OPTION 2: Get cheesy! Sprinkle on freshly grated hard cheese, like Parmesan, Romano, or Asiago before baking.

SNACKS

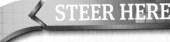

STEER HERE

SALTY SNACKS

KAIA SEA SALT & VINEGAR PUMPKIN SEEDS

- Organic - Sprouted

Also try their Garlic Sea Salt sunflower seeds.

BLUE MOUNTAIN EXTREME NUT MIX

- Organic - Sprouted - Nine types of nuts

Numerous varieties of sprouted nuts and seeds available.

JACKSON'S HONEST POTATO CHIPS

- Organic potatoes - Unrefined sea salt - Organic spices
- Organic coconut oil - Non-GMO

DANIELLE ROYAL SWEET POTATO CHIP

- Palm oil   *Also try their mango, pineapple, carrot, okra, and pumpkin chips.*
Beware: the coconut chips do contain sugar.

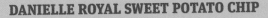

TRADER JOE'S ORGANIC POPCORN WITH OLIVE OIL

- Organic popcorn - Organic extra-virgin olive oil

ALIVE AND RADIANT QUITE CHEEZY KALE KRUNCH

- Organic kale - Sprouted cashew - Organic spices

Numerous varieties . . . we love the Southwest Ranch

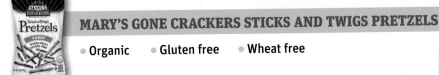

MARY'S GONE CRACKERS STICKS AND TWIGS PRETZELS

- Organic - Gluten free - Wheat free

LYDIA'S ORGANICS ITALIAN CRACKERS

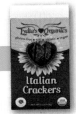

- Organic - Sprouted seeds and flax - Gluten free - Wheat free

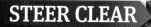

STEER CLEAR

SALTY SNACKS

BLUE DIAMOND WALNUTS

They're not sprouted, but the even bigger problem is that these nuts are coated in GMO corn oil and BHT (Banned Bad Boy preservative). The contents in the see-through bag appear to be only nuts; however, two added Poor Food ingredients are lurking.

DORITOS 100-CALORIE NACHO CHEESE TORTILLA CHIPS

This portion-controlled mini bag may save you from eating more than you want to, but it serves up a heavy load of Poor Food ingredients. The first three should all scream GMO to you—corn, vegetable oil, and maltodextrin (from corn). If that didn't make you put this "diet" snack back, maybe the nonorganic rBGH dairy products, three counterfeit colors, three forms of MSG, and vitamin C–depleting sugar will. And who are we really kidding? Our goal is to stop putting junk in our mouths, not choose smaller bags of it.

BOLD PARTY BLEND CHEX MIX

You'll be the pooper of the party when you serve this BHT-preserved cereal as a snack. Start with a heaping, belly-bloating bowl of refined wheat, add in corn meal (GMO), vegetable oil (GMO), sugar (EMD), MSG, maltodextrin (GMO), mono-glycerides (tricky trans fat), corn syrup solids (GMO), soy sauce (GMO), and corn flour (GMO), and coat it all with some extra wheat starch. Don't take this Chex mix to the checkout.

SENSIBLE PORTIONS VEGGIE STRAWS OR CHIPS

Can't get your kids to eat their veggies? Well, they will definitely love these tuber straws (i.e., potato chips) disguised to look like crudités (vegetable sticks). We bet they'll eat the whole bag. Unsuspecting parents won't know that these "veg-gie" snacks are made from potato flour (potato flakes and potato starch), sun-flower oil, wheat starch, sugar, and nonorganic turmeric. Where are the veggies? They're listed right in the ingredients . . . tomato puree and spinach powder—each with an insignificant contribution to the total calories and nutritional value of this Poor Food product.

SNACKS

RICH FOOD 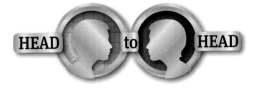 POOR FOOD

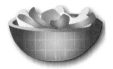
HEAD to **HEAD**

Homemade Veggie Chip Flip made with one organic zucchini, one cup of organic kale, and one medium carrot with one-and-a-half tablespoons of coconut oil.

One single-serving bag of Sensible Portions Veggie Chips.

146 / 60	Calories/calories from fat	130 / 60
120% DV	Vitamin C	20% DV
8% DV—that is 400% more	Iron	2% DV
400% DV	Vitamin A	0% DV
12% DV	Calcium	0% DV
700% DV	Vitamin K	0% DV
Metabolism-boosting coconut oil	Oil	Heat-processed sunflower oil
None added	Sugar	Added EMD sugar
None added	Wheat	Wheat belly
Unrefined sea salt and organic spices	Spices	Irradiated free-radical promoting

The homemade Veggie Chip Flips supply far more micronutrients.

The bag of potato starch-, sugar-, and vegetable powder-covered chips supply few micronutrients and numerous Poor Food ingredients.

Sweet

SALTY NOT YOUR THING? Do you crave cookies, ice cream, and chocolate? Just because a food is sweet doesn't make it off-limits. Here, we show you what you can make in your kitchen from all the healthy Rich Food ingredients you now have stocked. And for those with no time (or inclination) to bake, we have you covered under Steer Here.

Cookies

There's nothing like warm cookies fresh out of the oven, and you don't have to give them up entirely. For an occasional treat, just switch out the the recipes' wheat flours for almond or coconut flours, swap the sugar for stevia, and trade the man-made GMO vegetable oils for creamy coconut oil or grass-fed butter, and you are in business!

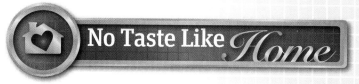

No Taste Like *Home*

For a change of pace from peanut butter, cash in with these delicious cashew butter cookies.

Better ~~Peanut~~ *Cashew* Butter Cookies

INGREDIENTS

- 1¼ cup sprouted cashew butter
- ½ tsp. baking soda
- ¼ cup (sprouted) almond flour
- ¼ cup coconut flour

- 2 large pastured eggs
- 1 tsp. pure vanilla extract
- ¼ tsp. pure stevia extract powder (equivalent to ½ cup of sugar). You can also use other sugar substitutes listed in Aisle 7.

DIRECTIONS

1 Preheat oven to 325 degrees.

2 Mix the ingredients in a bowl.

3 Spoon cookies using a tablespoon onto a butter-greased baking sheet.

4 Flatten cookies using a fork to make the traditional crosshatch peanut butter cookie design.

5 Bake for 20 minutes; look for crisping along rim.

6 Allow to cool before storing.

Ice Cream

You might literally run screaming from ice cream if you knew how EMD-filled most brands really are.

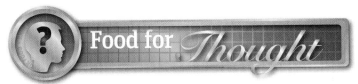
Food for *Thought*

Remember, ice cream starts with dairy, and unfortunately, most dairy contains synthetic hormones and antibiotics. Conventional cartons don't use grass-fed dairy, either, so purchasing them compromises our Rich Food milk and cream standards. While some may use real fruit, maybe even organic fruits for flavor, most rely on natural and imitation flavors and colors to create the thousands of varieties filling your grocer's freezer.

Here are a few of the common ice cream flavoring agents, descriptively called "natural flavors" or "artificial flavors" on labels.

NUT-FLAVORED ICE CREAM: Can come from butyraldehyde, an ingredient in rubber cement.

BANANA-FLAVORED ICE CREAM: Can come from amyl acetate, which is also used as an oil paint solvent.

PINEAPPLE-FLAVORED ICE CREAM: Can come from ethyl acetate, which is used as a leather or textile cleaner as well as in glues and nail polish removers.

CHERRY-FLAVORED ICE CREAM: Can come from aldehyde C17, an inflammable liquid used in synthetic dyes, plastic, and rubber.

And this one is not for those with weak stomachs....

VANILLA-, STRAWBERRY-, AND RASPBERRY-FLAVORED ICE CREAMS: Can include castoreum, a pus that oozes out of the castor sacs (located under the skin between the pelvis and the base of the tail) of mature beavers. We repeat: pus from a beaver's precious privates!

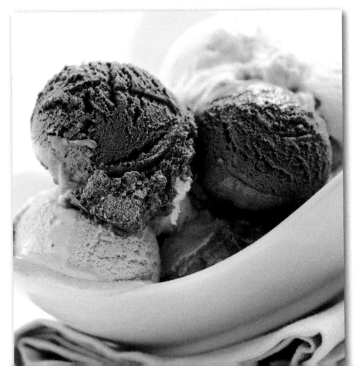

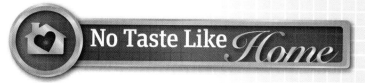

No Taste Like *Home*

You don't have to give up something you love in order to be healthy. Purchasing an ice cream maker is a fun investment, especially if you fancy frequent frozen fixes. See our favorites in our Rich Food Resource Center Online.

Creamy Coconut Ice Cream

INGREDIENTS

- 2 cans coconut milk (see our Rich Food options on page 60)
- 4 large pastured egg yolks (separate and discard the whites)
- 2 tsp. pure vanilla extract (see shopping guide on page 221)
- Pure stevia extract or alternative sweetener to taste

DIRECTIONS

1 Whisk eggs.

2 Add coconut milk and whisk again.

3 Pour into a medium saucepan and stir on medium heat until liquid thickens. Can take up to 10 minutes. Do not boil.

4 Remove from heat and cool.

5 Add vanilla and stevia and mix.

6 Place the liquid in your ice cream maker and follow manufacturer's instructions.

OPTION 1: Add unsweetened cocoa powder for a chocolaty coconut concoction.

OPTION 2: Go crazy! Add in a sink full of delicious mix-ins like sprouted nuts, unsweetened coconut flakes, or fresh organic berries.

OPTION 3: Make it raw! Replace the four eggs with four tablespoons of chia seeds soaked in one cup of water for thirty minutes. Blend with all of the other ingredients, and place in ice cream maker per manufacturer's instructions.

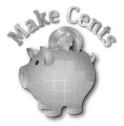

Is an ice cream maker not in your budget? Try our Yo'Pops. Simply blend organic Greek yogurt, stevia extract, and fresh berries until smooth, and pour mixture into Dixie cups. Insert a Popsicle stick in each cup, and place your batch in the freezer until solid (approximately five hours). Flip over and remove the Yo'Pop for a quick, delicious dessert. Tip: if you want to compete with the ice cream man, layer different berry blends in the cups.

Chocolate Bars

They may taste good, but we all know that these nutty, fudgy, sugary, low-quality chocolate bars aren't going to contribute to your micronutrient totals. Yes, even the dark chocolate varieties! In fact, the sugar and corn syrup in just about every store-bought bar will spike your insulin and send you plummeting to an irritable low. The sugar will block micronutrient absorption, lowering your immunity and tempting all forms of illness to set in.

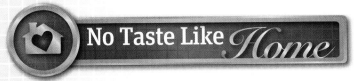

Mira's father, Burt, used to eat a ton of bittersweet chocolate bark, which is loaded with sugar. We set Burt straight with this Rich Food bark recipe, which is sugar-free and loaded with magnesium. The product gets its name because its rough, irregular texture resembles the bark of a tree—and because anyone who tries it barks for more!

Burt's Dark Chocolate Bark

INGREDIENTS

- 1 Tbsp. sugar-free dark cocoa powder (see Rich Food suggestions on page 214)
- 5 Tbsp. organic extra-virgin coconut oil
- 8 ounces of Baker's unsweetened 100 percent chocolate or similar
- 1 Tbsp. heavy organic whipping cream (preferably unpasteurized)
- ½ tsp. pure vanilla extract
- Stevia, or alternative sugar substitute of choice, to taste
- Pinch of unrefined sea salt
- 4 ounces sprouted nuts or seeds of your choice, chopped into small pieces

DIRECTIONS

1 Line a baking sheet or pan with wax paper or tinfoil.

2 Melt coconut oil in a small saucepan.

3 Add in cocoa and chocolate block and stir.

4 Add in cream and sweetener and blend well.

5 Stir in your nuts, seeds, or dried fruits.

6 Pour the mixture onto prepared surface; refrigerate for twenty minutes.

7 Break up bark into pieces and enjoy!

Store in the refrigerator.

OPTION #1: Add some unsweetened coconut flakes.

OPTION #2: Pour into fun-shaped mini ice cube trays to create individual chocolate snacks instead. They look elegant and are lovely to serve with coffee to create instant mochas.

STEER HERE

COOKIES

ALIVE & RADIANT ORIGINAL RAWEO COOKIES

- Organic • Soaked nuts • Naturally sweetened with raw honey

Also available in Oh So Fudgie and chai flavors.
Their Luscious Lemon Swirl is also a Rich Food option.

ICE CREAM

SO DELICIOUS NO SUGAR ADDED DAIRY FREE FROZEN DESSERTS

- Naturally sweetened with stevia and sugar alcohol
- Still contains gums and carrageenan

This is best option currently in the grocery store. Available in five flavors.

COCONUT SECRET MADAGASCAR VANILLA RAW COCONUT CREAM NON DAIRY DESSERT

- Naturally sweetened with coconut nectar
- Still contains thickeners

It isn't perfect, but for store-bought, it is a great option.

FRUIT BARS

LYDIA'S ORGANIC TROPICAL MANGO BAR

- Organic fruit • Sweetener free

Available in numerous fruit flavors.

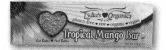

SNACKS

CANDY BARS

LUCIENNE'S SUGAR FREE 83% DARK CHOCOLATE BAR

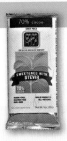

- Naturally sweetened with stevia

Dark, delicious, and soy free.

COCO POLO 70% COCOA DARK CHOCOLATE BAR

- Non-GMO ingredients
- Naturally sweetened with stevia and sugar alcohol
- Still contains soy in the form of non-GMO soy lecithin

Available in numerous dark chocolate and milk chocolate flavors.

RAWMIO ORGANIC SPROUTED HAZELNUT & FIG CHOCOLATE BARK

- Organic
- Raw sprouted hazelnuts
- Himalayan salt
- Naturally sweetened with coconut sugar

COOKIES

WHONU 2X STUFFED COOKIES

Whonu, indeed. Who knew that you could try to tout cookies as nutritious by tossing vitamins into unbelievably bad ingredients. The first ingredient in these "nutritious" snacks is sugar (EMD), followed by wheat (ADHD warning), polydextrose (GMO), soybean and canola oils (GMO), mono and diglycerides (trans fats), dextrose, corn syrup and yellow corn flour (GMO and EMDs), soy lecithin (GMO), and, of course, natural and artificial flavors (MSG). Whatever vitamins were stuffed into this batch of bad guys will be poorly assimilated by the body, thanks to the destructive effects of all these chemicals and digestion and immune-compromising Poor Food ingredients. Yes, kids need their vitamins, but not at the expense of all of these Poor Food ingredients.

ICE CREAM

BREYERS BLAST COOKIES AND CREAM MINT ICE CREAM

This frozen dessert adds in sixteen Poor Food ingredients. Sugar appears four times on the ingredient list. There are trans fats from mono and diglycerides, and numerous ingredients are GMO regulars, like canola oil, corn syrup, and soybean oil. They top off this dessert with artificial colors, EMD thickeners, and gums. Parents beware—none of the Breyers flavors did much better than this one.

SKINNY COW CHOCOLATE FUDGE BROWNIE ICE CREAM

This skinny cow could make you a sickly cow. The first three ingredients are non-organic skim milk (rBGH), sugar (EMD), and corn syrup (GMO/EMD). The brownie includes wheat (great for belly bloat!), GMO corn syrup, and hunger-inducing MSG flavoring. And this frozen skimmed concoction is thickened with three types of cellulose, GMO soy lecithin, one gum, one emulsifier, and carrageenan (MSG).

CANDY BARS

3 MUSKETEERS BAR

They may have been friends, but there is nothing friendly about this bar. When you chomp down on one of these airy nougat bars, you add 40 grams of sugar to your day. That is nearly double the amount of sugar of the daily recommendation for women by the American Heart Association! Even splitting the bar among three friends delivers too much Poor Food!

SNACKS

□ Choose soaked/sprouted nuts and seeds.

□ Choose chips in palm, coconut, or olive oil.

□ Choose organic chips when the bases are on the Terrible Twenty.

□ Choose sea vegetables for a micronutrient-rich alternative.

□ Avoid chocolate made with sugar and high fructose corn syrup.

□ Choose organic ice cream to avoid growth hormones and antibiotics in dairy.

□ Avoid cookies that contain wheat, sugar, or vegetable oils.

My go-to Rich Food choices for snacks: _____

_____

_____

_____

_____

_____

_____

_____

_____

_____

_____

_____

_____

_____

_____

_____

Aisle NINE

· ·

Beverages

The last aisle we turn down on our grocery expedition is the beverage aisle, where the drink you choose can either healthfully hydrate you or seriously sabotage your health. Even when buying every Rich Food option in the supermarket, the beverage aisle is where many otherwise smart shoppers backslide in their quest for micronutrient sufficiency. That is because one of the biggest problems plaguing the beverage aisle can be summed up in one little word—*sugar*.

While the word may be little, there is nothing small about the amount of excess sugar Americans are consuming. According to the American Heart Association (AHA), the average child between four and eight consumes seven times more than the recommended maximum daily sugar allowance. That's around twenty-one teaspoons of extra sugar a day! Fourteen- to eighteen-year-olds take more than five times their recommended allowance—a whopping thirty-four teaspoons. And adults consume less than the American teenager, averaging twenty-two teaspoons a day, but that's still at least four times the amount the AHA says adults should have for good health.

What if we told you that of the total sugar adults and children consume, approximately 50 percent of it comes from beverages?! That's right, we are drinking ourselves into an abyss of obesity and disease. Remember, excess sugar in any form has negative health implications. First, it causes a sudden jump in blood sugar, which signals the body to release the fat storage hormone insulin. In this way, excess sugar can contribute to fat

243

accumulation and also inhibit your ability to burn stored body fat. If this happens repeatedly over time, the body can become insulin resistant, which can lead to type 2 diabetes. Additionally, sugar can cause chromium and copper deficiencies, block the absorption of calcium and magnesium, and compete with vitamin C for cell receptor sites on white blood cells. When vitamin C enters those receptor sites, it can help build a strong immune system. However, when sugar supersedes, it restricts vitamin C from entering, and the immune system can be greatly compromised.

With all of these complications arising from drinking sugar-laden beverages, it would seem as if you might be better off putting down the bottles altogether. However, you still need to drink something. After all, hydration is extremely important. Your body is just over 50 percent water, and it needs to stay that way. We don't want you to boycott the beverages—we just need to implement a little Rich Food reasoning when choosing them.

• • • • • • • • • • • • • • • • • • • •

Soda

SO, WHAT IS SO WRONG WITH SODA? Let's see . . . oh, *everything!* While we could go on for pages on the sins of soda, we will spare you. Instead, here are our top ten reasons to avoid soda.

1 Sugar (EMD)—For even more information on sugar, pick up *Naked Calories* and flip to page 104.

2 High fructose corn syrup (HFCS—EMD).

3 Caramel color and other counterfeit colors (possible carcinogens and may cause hyperactivity in children).

4 Phosphoric acid (EMD).

5 Artificial flavors (MSG).

6 Sodium benzoate (possible carcinogen).

7 Brominated vegetable oil (BBB).

8 Artificial sweeteners (SSS).

9 Calcium disodium EDTA (mineral-leaching EMD).

10 High levels of acid (citric, tartaric, malic, etc.)—erodes tooth enamel. Most soda has a pH level of 2, which is one hundred thousand times more acidic than a neutral pH of 7.

This is far from a complete list, but soda is the epitome of Poor Food. Soda doesn't provide any nutrition, and what's worse, it actually leaves you more micronutrient depleted when you are done drinking it. Yep, you're actually worse off because there are four EMD ingredients in soda that deplete you of essential micronutrients your body already has from eating Rich Foods. So when

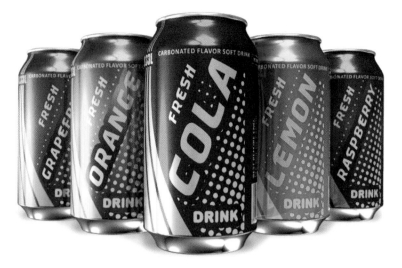

you take out all ten of those nasty ingredients, your soda, pop, or soft drink is nothing more than a simple glass of carbonated soda water—a much healthier choice, in our opinion.

While there are numerous reasons to vilify soda, carbonation is not one. We hate to burst anyone's bubble here—but carbonation itself *does not* leach calcium, harm teeth, or cause damage to your stomach. The aforementioned Poor Food ingredients are to blame. So, drinking a soda water with a splash of lemon or lime can serve up all the refreshment with none of the guilt.

Are diet sodas any better? Not really. While they do get rid of the sugar and HFCS, they still contain everything else on the list—especially number eight, the Sinister Sugar Substitutes. What's more, some studies have shown that people who drink diet sodas actually have larger waist circumferences, suffer more strokes and heart attacks, and have higher blood sugar levels and increased risk of diabetes than those who don't. Therefore, drinking a diet soda may save you from the calories, but not the adverse health consequences of soda consumption.

Energy and Sports Drinks

THE ENERGY AND SPORTS DRINK market is exploding, but these two categories of "healthy" drinks can be dangerously deceiving, because even those who *never* drink soda will sometimes drink energy or sports drinks and think nothing of it. Energy drinks are nothing more than soda with extra caffeine and a few micronutrients of dubious bio-availability thrown in for good marketing. Sports drinks are simply non-carbonated, artificially colored sugar waters with electrolytes, sodium and potassium, thrown in for good measure. A glance at the label reveals that some of these drinks contain less overall sugar than traditional sodas, but they can become highly addictive. Further, the diet or sugar-free versions are often full of Poor Food Sinister Sugar Substitutes. If you are looking for energy, we suggest coffee or tea, and because of its naturally high potassium levels, coconut water is a great-tasting sports drink alternative.

Juice

IF WE HAD A DOLLAR for every time someone asked us what we thought about juice . . . well, let's just say we wish we did. Yes, juice is natural*ish*, in the sense that you make it by squeezing a piece of fruit to extract juice. However, juice absent of its natural covering, i.e., the fruit, can quickly become a high-calorie, high-sugar, insulin-spiking beverage that doesn't satiate as well as eating the actual fruit.

Additionally, in all of our six years of travel to more than 135 countries, we never witnessed a remote group or tribe that woke up and enjoyed a tall glass of juice for breakfast. Fruit—yes; coconut water—yes; freshly squeezed exotic Amazon or Tibetan fruit juice—no. While a glass of your favorite juice now and again is not the end of the world, we urge you instead to consume your fruits whole. This will moderate your overall amount of sugar ingestion and maximize micronutrient intake. Remember, local seasonal fruits are best because they have traveled the least distance.

If you still feel that breakfast wouldn't be the same without that tall glass of juice to wash it down, then here are some guidelines to help you identify which juices are the most judicious. The gold standard for juice is to be labeled "100 percent juice." However, don't be misled by this first-class promise, either, because while the beverage may be from pure juice, there is no guarantee that it isn't watered down, or that citric acid or artificial flavors or colors have not been added in. It is time to divide and conquer again, as it is only by reading the ingredients that you will see what has been mixed in to the 100 percent pure juice.

Now, it may surprise you to learn that according to the Centers for Disease Control and Prevention (CDC), "about 98 percent of all juices sold in the United States are pasteurized." Hey, wait a second—an EMD just snuck into the carton of juice! Juice is pasteurized the same way milk is pasteurized and for the same reasons, meaning that your store-bought juice has undergone the same micronutrient-depleting heat treatment as your milk in order to extend its shelf life. This is true for all juices, including concentrates. And if you have always wondered the difference between juices labeled "not from concentrate" and those "from concentrates," here's the deal. Juices that are "from concentrates" often cost less, as they save manufacturers money. Concentrating entails that the water be removed from the juice. This ensures that juice producers have less waste and can freeze what they cannot immediately sell. By removing the water, this concentrated juice can be inexpensively shipped around the world, further advancing their profits. When the water is removed, what remains is "concentrated" fruit sugar. A carton of "juice from concentrate" contains fresh water that has been added to that concentrated fruit sugar. Voilà—you have a more processed, less natural, higher-margin juice.

Then there are fruit juices labeled "punch," "cocktail," "splash," or "drink," which are really food industry code words for "fake juice." As if 100 percent pure fruit juice is not flavorful, sweet, or brightly colored enough, some companies who should know better surreptitiously fill their bottles with Poor Food ingredients. Take Campbell's V8 Splash, one of the healthiest-sounding juices at the store. This product contains high fructose corn syrup, 10 percent fruit and vegetable concentrates (pure sugar), counterfeit color red #40, and the Sinister Sugar Substitute sucralose. Then they splash a label on it (in this case, V8 Splash) touting high antioxidant content and a certification by the American Heart Association applauding the low levels of saturated fat and cholesterol. But think about it—when has any natural juice ever had saturated fat or cholesterol to begin with . . . unless it's not an all-natural juice beverage? Certified "healthy" beverages like these are masquerading as safe, juice-like drinks for your family.

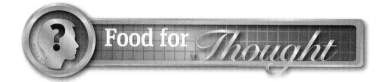

To get the most out of the juice you do drink, we recommend freshly squeezed, unpasteurized juice, diluted with water to reduce the sugar content. Keep in mind the Terrible Twenty when deciding which juice you need to purchase organic. Tip: you may want to consider a probiotic juice. Some companies are fermenting juice, which supplies live, active bacteria to support immune and digestive health.

Coffee and Tea

COFFEE AND TEA are often categorized together, but did you know that except for water, tea is the most commonly consumed beverage in the world? The first reference of tea use traces as far back as the tenth century BC. Coffee, on the other hand, is a newcomer to the beverage arena, invented in the seventeenth century AD. However, coffee has come a long way in the past few centuries. Along with soda and beer, coffee ranks right behind tea as one of the world's most consumed beverages. While most of us enjoy one or both of these beverages on a regular basis, many are unsuspecting of their terrific health benefits.

Coffee, for example, is the number one source of antioxidants in the US diet, and by a mile. It contains 300 percent more antioxidants than black tea and 3,333 percent more than an apple! Antioxidants have been shown to prevent free radicals from causing damage to cells. Additionally, antioxidant consumption has been shown to reduce the risk of heart disease, depression, Alzheimer's, Parkinson's, type 2 diabetes, strokes, cirrhosis of the liver, gout, dementia, and certain types of cancer.

To be fair, caffeine is an EMD due to its slight depletion of calcium. It can cause jitteriness and headaches if consumed in excess. Adding a dollop of calcium-rich dairy or occasionally choosing decaf coffee and tea to balance an insatiable coffee/tea habit might be helpful in decreasing the incidence of such side effects. Caffeine also contains several polyphenols that can inhibit the absorption of non-heme iron, which could lead to iron-deficiency anemia. Additionally, research has shown that coffee consumption can increase the risk of acid reflux.

So here is the bottom line: for thousands of years, tea has been used as a health tonic, and it can be enjoyed daily. Regarding coffee, Frank Hu, MD, MPH, PhD, nutrition and epidemiology professor at the Harvard School of Public Health, says, "There is certainly much more good news than bad news, in terms of coffee and health."

We think these brews are safe bets!

Coffee

Coffee beans are really the seeds of a coffee berry, from a coffea plant native to tropical and southern Africa and tropical Asia. Ironically, while the coffee plant is not native to Brazil, Brazil is currently the largest producer of coffee (2,874,310 tons a year) with Vietnam, Indonesia, Colombia, and India rounding out the top five. According to the Mayo Clinic, an average eight-ounce cup of coffee contains between 95 and 200 mg of caffeine. A coffee's color, boldness, and caffeine content is determined by how long a coffee seed (bean) is roasted. The longer the roast, the bolder the flavor, the darker the color, and the more caffeine the coffee loses. So the next time you order a bold coffee, don't assume that also means the beverage will embolden your attention span. Blond roast, the light-colored coffee, retains more of its natural caffeine.

Even with all the health benefits and the tremendous variety of tastes, colors, and blends coffee delivers, it may be the heaviest chemically treated food commodity in the world. The synthetic petroleum-based fertilizers commonly used in coffee production slowly destroy soil fertility and contaminate local water supplies. Buying organic coffee reduces the global use of these synthetic fertilizers and sends a message that you care about clean water, clean soil, and healthy beverages.

To make matters worse, coffee's popularity is accelerating the rate of global deforestation. Coffee trees naturally grow in the shade of a dense rainforest. To increase productivity, however, nearly 70 percent of the world's coffee production now comes from sun-resistant coffee tree hybrids. Deforestation occurs as growers make way for more sun-resistant coffee trees. Again, buying organic is preferred because most organic coffee has been "shade grown."

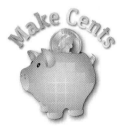

Think about buying coffee with the "fair trade" label. Using this label requires a certification process, and it indicates that the grower paid a fair wage to laborers. Think of "fair trade" as being to local economies and its workers what "organic" is to the environment and food. While fair trade coffee may cost you a bit more, you are paying it forward by supporting fair wages for workers in developing countries.

Teas

Here is a short reference guide to *tea-ch* you about teas and their individual benefits.

Pu'erh

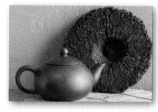

THE CHOLESTEROL CURE. Grown exclusively in and around Pu'erh in Yunnan Province, China, pu'erh teas are aged, fermented, and traditionally molded into birdnest-like forms and are known for significantly improving blood cholesterol levels. One study done at the Wun-Shan Branch Tea Research and Extension Station in Taipei, Taiwan, showed that pu'erh tea leaves caused both an increase of HDL (good cholesterol) and a decrease in LDL ("bad" cholesterol). Enjoy a fine, aged cup of this ancient cholesterol cure today.

Black (including Earl Grey)

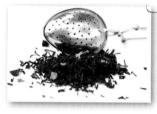

MINIMIZE THE MUFFIN TOP. The most popular teas in the Western world, black teas, are traditionally from China, India, and Sri Lanka (Ceylon). A study from University College London revealed that study participants who drank black tea after a stressful event were found to have almost 50 percent lower levels of the stress hormone cortisol in their blood. And remember, elevated cortisol levels promote an increase in stubborn stomach fat. Drinking this black beauty can help you to say bye-bye to belly fat.

Oolong

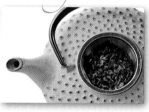

OXIDIZE WITH OOLONG! All oolong teas come from China or Taiwan and are highly favored and desired amongst tea connoisseurs. It is highly studied for its metabolism-boosting effects. In a study at the US Agricultural Research Services' Diet and Human Laboratory, participants increased fat oxidation (fat burning) by a whOOping 12 percent after consuming oolong tea versus caffeinated water. This tea's powerful caffeine and antioxidants put your fat-burning engine into overdrive.

Green

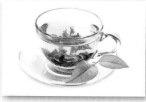

A CALORIE-BURNING MACHINE. A green tea signifies that the leaf was heated immediately after plucking, which preserves it from withering and oxidation. Green tea has a natural green color (hence the name) and more tannins (EMD), vitamin C, minerals, and chlorophyll than either oolong or black tea. Hence, green tea has a more astringent taste, leaving that familiar sharp aftertaste sensation. Japanese scientists determined that the green tea's *epigallocatechin gallate* (EGCG) induces thermogenesis, an internal heating process that increases calorie burn. In studies, drinking three cups of green tea daily was shown to burn an extra two hundred fifty calories a day—enough to lose twenty-five pounds a year. Go green and get lean!

White

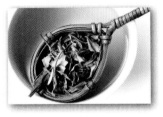

SAGGY OR SMOOTH? Mostly grown in the Fujian Province of China, white tea gets its name from the fine silvery-white hairs on the unopened buds of the tea plant, which have been steamed and dried. This minimally processed tea inhibits the activity of the enzymes elastase and collagenase, which break down the proteins elastin and collagen in the body. Both proteins are essential to maintain the elasticity of skin. So, when you drink white, it will help you stay tight!

Herbal "Tea"

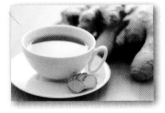

HEAPS OF HEALTH. You may have noticed herbal "teas" in your grocery store and wondered how they were different from regular teas. Interestingly, these herbal infusions are not tea at all in that they do not contain any tea leaves (from tea plants). Instead, these 100 percent caffeine-free beverages are often combinations of well-known herbs such as chamomile, ginger, lemongrass, lavender, licorice, and others, which deliver a variety of health benefits as well as an enjoyable adventure of aromatherapy and flavor. While ginger tea staves off seasickness, you can try chamomile for calming, or lemon balm to boost concentration. Milk thistle and dandelion teas work to detoxify and regenerate the liver, and rosehip tea supplies an abundance of immunity-boosting vitamin C.

Yerba Mate

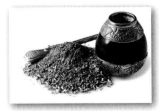

MELLOW INTENSITY. Sipped in South America out of hollow calabash gourds through a silver straw called a bombilla, mate is actually a species of holly plant first introduced to the world by the Guaraní Indians in modern-day Paraguay and Argentina. It is high in vitamin C, magnesium, manganese, and potassium and also contains three members of the xanthine family: caffeine, theobromine, and theophylline. Together this trio acts quite differently in the body than caffeine alone and is described as producing a relaxing effect while enhancing one's alertness and focus. It gives you an up that is downright dreamy.

Water

YOU WOULDN'T THINK there would be much difficulty in choosing water, but just like everything else in the grocery store, there is Rich Food water and Poor Food water. And why do we buy bottled water anyway? While it may seem like bottled water is a relatively new phenomenon, we have actually been bottling spring water for its therapeutic minerals since the late 1700s. Of course, water used to be bottled in glass bottles, while today the good majority is bottled in plastic for convenience and cost savings. While we all know that plastic bottles are not healthy for us or the environment, the number on the bottom of the bottle can help us choose bottles made from plastic that is the least offensive for both. (See page 33 for more info on BPA and plastics.)

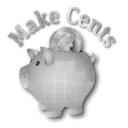

Don't want to spend money on bottled water but are still concerned about the quality of your family's drinking water? Perhaps investing in a water filter would be the best way to ensure clean, great-tasting water at home. But how do you know if you need a water filter, or how to tell which of the hundreds of filters on the market is best? Start by determining the quality of water in your municipality. How? Call the EPA's Safe Drinking Water Hotline (800-426-4791) for the names of state-certified testing labs or for your local health authority—they might even offer low-cost or free test kits. Also check out epa.gov/safewater/labs. You may ultimately find that you don't need a water filter at all. However, if you do, your next step is to choose a filter that will meet your purifying needs as well as your family's quantity demand. ConsumerReports.org is a good place to start evaluating products, and there is probably a specialty supplier in your area that can provide a free in-home consultation.

Flavored and Vitamin Waters

Flavored waters are bottled in sparkling and flat varieties and in the form of the ever-popular, make-it-yourself, flavor packets like Crystal Light. These beverages can be nightmares comprised of sugar or multiple SSS, citric acid (a little is okay, but too much can really lower pH and cause enamel erosion), maltodextrin, artificial flavors, every artificial color under the carcinogenic rainbow, and BHA. Choose flavored waters with just water and natural flavors and avoid those that add in the plethora of Poor Food ingredients.

Next, there are the super popular and somewhat confusing waters that add in vitamins. While at first glance these waters seem like they would be a healthy option, they're not. In fact, the Center for Science in the Public Interest (CSPI) has brought a lawsuit against Coca-Cola over what the CSPI says are deceptive and unsubstantiated claims by Coca-Cola about their Vitaminwater line of soft drinks. While you may not think of vitamin-enhanced waters as soft drinks, here is what Steve Gardner, litigation director for CSPI, had to say on the subject:

> For too long, Coca-Cola has been exploiting Americans' desire to eat and drink more healthfully by deceiving them into thinking that Vitaminwater can actually prevent disease. In fact, Vitaminwater is no more than non-carbonated soda, providing unnecessary added sugar and contributing to weight gain, obesity, diabetes, and other diseases.

Coke's lawyers fired back, making the incredible statement that no reasonable person could possibly conclude Vitaminwater was a healthy beverage! From the front, these "water" beverages look like nothing more than lightly flavored, vitamin-infused water, but when we apply our divide-and-conquer philosophy and turn these bottles around, we quickly see that products like Vitaminwater, Vidration, SoBe Lifewater, Dasani vitamin-enhanced waters, and many others are nothing more than Poor Food ingredients packaged to trick us.

Coconut Water

A newbie to the performance drink market is coconut water. While some enjoy the flavor of coconut water, others find it to be an acquired taste. So is coconut water a Rich Food or a Poor Food? Well, that depends. There have been plenty of days when we were hiking for miles through hot rainforests and were very happy to have one of our guides chop off the top of a coconut and hand it to us. This natural, delicious, micronutrient-dense liquid is obviously a Rich Food.

But what about the coconut water in the grocery store? While it is probable that it has lost some of its original essential micronutrients on its long trip from jungle to market, pure coconut water is still a Rich Food, bursting with electrolytes such as potassium and magnesium. However, we should caution that although it is natural, coconut water is similar to juice in that it still contains a lot of insulin-spiking sugar. So while coconut water can be a great substitute for sports drinks during or after heavy exercise, or during a long day in the sun, you may not want to guzzle it like water. And watch out for some of the sugar-laden coconut water concoctions. These hybrids are good examples of Poor Food distortions of the real thing encased inside its tough shell.

STEER HERE

SODA

ZEVIA ALL NATURAL SODA - MOUNTAIN ZEVIA FLAVOR

- GMO free   • No phosphoric acid
- Sweetened with stevia and sugar alcohol

Beware: some flavors contain caramel color.

JUICE

LAKEWOOD ORGANIC PURE APPLE JUICE

- Organic   • Nothing but apple juice   • Not from concentrate

Many juice varieties available under their Pure label.

UNCLE MATT'S ORGANIC ORANGE JUICE

- Organic   • BPA-free packaging   • Just the juice

Also available in other juice varieties.

KEVITA COCONUT SPARKLING PROBIOTIC DRINK

- Organic   • Four strands of live cultures
- Naturally sweetened with stevia   • Low-calorie
- Low sugar content

Your tummy will thank you. The Living Greens and Lemon Ginger flavors are made with organic cane syrup—best to opt for the other flavors.

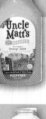

ZUKAY BEET GINGER KVASS

- Organic ingredients   • Probiotic active cultures   • Raw
- Low sugar content

Also try the other incredible probiotic combinations.

BEVERAGES

COFFEE AND TEA

CAMANO ISLAND COFFEE FROM PAPUA NEW GUINEA (MEDIUM ROAST)

- Organic
- Fair trade certified
- Shade grown

PUBLIX GREENWISE MARKET COFFEE

- Organic
- Fair trade certified

Available in French Roast, Columbian, and Breakfast Blend.

CAFFE NATURAL ANTIOXIDANT COFFEE

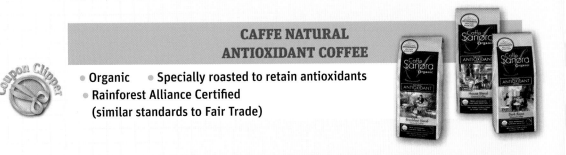

- Organic
- Specially roasted to retain antioxidants
- Rainforest Alliance Certified (similar standards to Fair Trade)

UPGRADED COFFEE BY THE BULLETPROOF EXECUTIVE

- Specially processed to prevent high mycotoxin (bad fungus) levels
- BPA-free packaging

ARBOR TEAS JASMINE GREEN TEA

- Organic
- Fair trade certified
- Co2 decaffeinated varieties

Many varieties available.

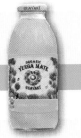

GUAYAKI UNSWEETENED YERBA MATE

- Organic
- Great tea beverage and energy drink

WATER

MOUNTAIN VALLEY SPRING WATER

- Glass bottles
- Purity NSF certified (NSF is the leading global provider of public health and safety-based risk management)

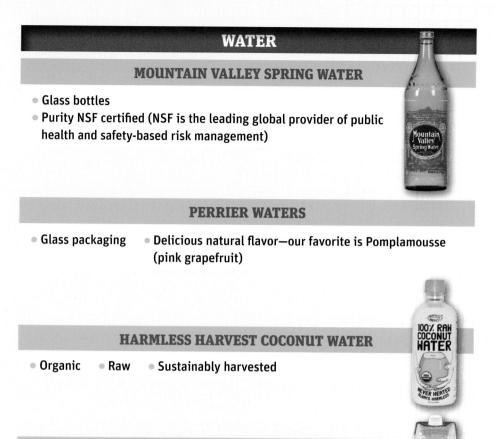

PERRIER WATERS

- Glass packaging
- Delicious natural flavor—our favorite is Pomplamousse (pink grapefruit)

HARMLESS HARVEST COCONUT WATER

- Organic
- Raw
- Sustainably harvested

VITA COCO PURE COCONUT WATER UNFLAVORED

- Sugar free and natural

SODA

MOUNTAIN DEW

The neon color alone should be enough to indicate this drink is not healthy. By combining sodium benzoate with vitamin C–rich orange juice concentrate, this product forms benzene, a known carcinogen, and regardless of how little is formed, why take the risk at all? Add in HFCS (GMO/EMD), mineral-leaching disodium EDTA, the Bad Banned Boy brominated vegetable oil, and Counterfeit Color yellow #5, and you should do yourself a favor and *don't do the Dew!*

JUICE

TAMPICO TROPICAL PUNCH

This punch is more like a slap in the face. Watered-down GMO micronutrient-depleting high fructose corn syrup mixed with juice solids and concentrates, modified food starch (GMO, MSG), EDTA (mineral-leaching EMD), and possible carcinogens potassium benzoate and red #40, drinking this tropical punch may put you down for the count.

SUNNY-D TANGY ORIGINAL

Have you ever seen the little candies that look like slices of fruit, but are made completely out of sugar? That is basically what Sunny-D is. Instead of 100 percent pure fruit juice, it's a water and corn syrup (EMD, GMO) beverage with modified cornstarch (GMO); canola oil (GMO); three sinister sugar substitiutes—sucralose, acesulfame potassium, and neotame; and also contains artificial colors yellow #5 and #6. It only contains 2 percent or less of real juice, in the form of non-organic apple (Terrible Twenty), orange, tangerine, lime, and grapefruit juice concentrates (sugar). We give this product a not so Sunny-"F." They couldn't even get their name right.

GATORADE G SERIES PERFORM CITRUS COOLER

What do you need after a tough workout? How about a plastic bottle filled with sugar? Slap a G on the label, pay big endorsement fees to famous athletes, and you have a recipe for a successful advertising campaign. Don't buy into the nonsense—no one needs to gulp down 56 grams of sugar from a 32-ounce bottle. It is loaded with yellow #6 and brominated vegetable oil, which are banned in other countries. Does this sound like a smart way to increase your athletic performance or replenish yourself after one? G . . . we don't think so.

CELESTIAL SEASONINGS GINKGO SHARP CRAN-FRUIT-BLEND ENERGY JUICE DRINK

With a name like Celestial Seasonings, it should be heavenly. Instead, what you get is high fructose corn syrup (EMD, GMO) with fruit juice concentrates, including both apples and strawberries from the Terrible Twenty. And if you finish this 20-ounce bottle, you also consume 85 grams of sugar—that's twenty-two teaspoons. That amount of sugar will take your waistline straight to hell.

CRYSTAL LIGHT FRUIT PUNCH

It may be light on calories but it is heavy in Poor Food ingredients. You will be serving your loved ones high levels of enamel-stripping citric acid, maltodextrin (sugar, GMO), aspartame and acesulfame potassium (two SSS), modified corn starch (GMO), artificial flavors (MSG), two counterfeit colors (red #40 and blue #1), and the Banned Bad Boy BHT in every chilled glass.

COFFEE AND TEA

STARBUCKS COFFEE FRAPPUCCINO

As if people didn't drink enough of Starbucks dessert coffee drinks at numerous locations, Starbucks has now made its way to your grocery store. This little honey is Starbucks coffee mixed with maltodextrin (sugar, GMO), pectin (EMD), and as much sugar (EMD) as *four* Little Debbie Honey Buns.

SOBE LIFEWATER WITH COCONUT WATER MANGO MANDARIN

Neither mangos nor mandarin oranges appear in the ingredients. What does? SoBe has taken filtered water and added in sugar (EMD) and coconut juice concentrate (more sugar). They top off the contents of their plastic bottles with caramel color and add in some stevia to insinuate it is a sugar-free beverage, which obviously it is not.

☐ Choose soda without the Ten Poor Food ingredients we listed.

☐ Choose coffee or tea as natural energy.

☐ Choose unsweetened coconut water as a natural sports drink alternative.

☐ Choose 100 percent pure juice not from concentrate without any added ingredients.

☐ Choose organic fair trade coffee and teas.

☐ Choose water in safe plastic bottles or glass bottles.

☐ Choose a good water filter for your home if needed.

☐ Avoid flavored waters with added Poor Food ingredients.

☐ Avoid drink mix packets with added artificial colors and sweeteners.

*My go-to Rich Food choices beverages:*_____

_____

_____

_____

_____

_____

Aisle TEN

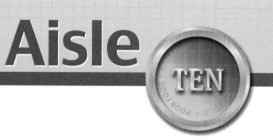

Checkout · Conclusion

Y ou now know how to discern a Rich Food from a Poor Food in every aisle of the grocery store—or anywhere else, for that matter. How many food items did you toss from your kitchen or avoid buying while you were reading this book? Many people tell us that large sections of their pantry are bare by the time they hit the beverage aisle. But most important, they tell us that the information they learned in *Rich Food, Poor Food* has completely changed the way they grocery shop! And we have to tell you, nothing could make us happier, because this is precisely why we wrote *Rich Food, Poor Food*. We wanted to create a forum to educate consumers as to what is really being put into the foods they are buying and to show them that there are healthy alternatives as long as they know what to look for.

You may have noticed that we didn't cover every single food in your grocery store. That's because *Rich Food, Poor Food* is not meant to be a guide you need to lean on every time you

259

want to know whether a food is rich or poor. Instead, we designed *Rich Food, Poor Food* to teach you how to quickly and decisively identify a Rich Food from a Poor Food on your own. After all, as the adage goes, "Give a man a fish, and you feed him for a day; teach a man to fish, and you feed him for a lifetime."

We know you are busy, so we are not going to take up too much more of your time now that the GPS has done its job and delivered you to a more micronutrient-sufficient destination. Here are the main points we hope you take away from our experience together.

You Have Arrived

 CHILL: If you feel overwhelmed right now, don't worry. As you use your *Rich Food, Poor Food* GPS frequently, the concepts and terminology will become more familiar. Before long, you will be sailing through the aisles, pointing out Poor Food ingredients to perfect strangers.

 DO YOUR BEST: No one expects you to be perfect. We know we're not! So if Poor Food ends up on your cart now and then, don't feel that you have failed. *Rich Food, Poor Food* offers guidelines, not orders. Use it to help you make better choices, not to make you feel guilty for being indulgent now and then.

 INVEST: Although it is true that some of the Rich Food choices can cost a little more than the Poor Food choices, you aren't just buying groceries anymore–you're buying Rich Food! You should be convinced by now that every extra penny you spend is an investment in your health. We can't think of a single thing more important to spend your hard-earned money on.

 SHARE: Share this important information with relatives, coworkers, teachers, and friends so that they too can improve their health by increasing the quality of foods that they eat every day. But remember, be a patient, nonjudgmental teacher. Not everyone has read *Rich Food, Poor Food* (even though we wish they would). Do not expect them to know what you know about every Poor Food ingredient.

 GET NAKED: If you haven't yet read *Naked Calories,* what are you waiting for? It will give you a much better understanding of how the Rich Food, Poor Food philosophy fits into our three-step approach to optimal health.

INDULGE: Start a love affair with Rich Food. Not only will it enhance your health, it will enhance your life. And if a particular food company has really impressed you, let them know. Starting a small food company or farm is not the fast track to fame and fortune. Being a visionary is often a thankless job.

 SPREAD THE WORD: Tell everyone to read *Rich Food, Poor Food*. And if you see that we are going to be speaking in your area (CaltonNutrition.com/upcoming-appearances.aspx), come and see us. We can't wait to meet you!

LIKE EVERY GREAT ADVENTURE, ours is coming to a close. But this isn't good-bye. Even if you can't make it to one of our appearances, visit us on the Web. We stocked our Rich Food Resource Center (RFRC) on CaltonNutriton.com/Rich-Food with all kinds of great tools for you to use. Remember the Coupon Clipper icons throughout the book? The RFRC is the place you will find all the money-saving coupons for some incredible Rich Food products that we have lined up for you. And more manufacturers are coming on board all the time to help make sure that everyone can afford to purchase Rich Food.

We want to hear from you. Let us know if you find a Rich Food option that we might have missed. (Like we said, we aren't perfect!) We will use your input to continually update our Rich Food Resource Center and highlight new food companies that are doing it right. We all have a long road ahead of us if we want to change the face of the current supermarket . . . but together, we can make a difference.

There are two more great tools awaiting you in the resource center as well. First, we have created a great eco-shopping tote designed not only to benefit the environment, but to help you navigate the grocery store safely by reminding you of some of our favorite tips from *Rich Food, Poor Food*. They are free* . . . while supplies last. Second, you will find a Grocery Store Rich Food Request List available for download. Simply print the list of our Rich Food choices, check off items you

*shipping and handling may apply

desire that your supermarket currently does not stock, and bring the list to your store managers. Let them know that you would like to purchase the Rich Foods on that list and ask them to please stock them for you.

It's not the managers' fault if they don't carry all the foods on the list (yet). However, it is your right and responsibility to let the management team at your grocery store know what you are looking for and the kind of food quality you expect. We have found that most stores are happy to accommodate Rich Food requests whenever possible—especially when numerous individuals work as a team and request the same foods. Imagine the impact we can all have on the quality of the products stocked on store shelves. We can literally crowd out Poor Foods simply by requesting that Rich Food options are stocked and collectively boycotting products that blatantly disregard human health.

And last, and perhaps most important, we want to say thank you for reading *Rich Food, Poor Food*. People like you make promoting good health worthwhile, and hey, at least now we won't be the only people in the grocery store reading the ingredient lists.

Healthy shopping!

M. Calton

Appendix One

Say No to GMOs

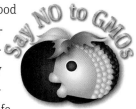

We love food, and we love the companies that prioritize food quality and safety. The manufacturers listed in this appendix do not use genetically modified organisms in the ingredients. The brand names labeled with an asterisk* are even third-party tested by the Non GMO Project to ensure the claims are accurate. Supporting manufacturers who say no to GMOs helps keep your family safe and sends a strong message to the stores about what nutrition standards should be adhered to. However, just because they are free of GMOs doesn't guarantee they are free of other Poor Food ingredients. Make sure to read the ingredients list for yourself to be sure.

Aisle 1: Dairy

YOU CAN BE ASSURED that these dairies don't use GMOs, even if they aren't labeled as organic:

Alta Dena Organics	Nancy's Organic Dairy*	Seven Stars Farm*
Butterworks Farm	Natural by Nature	Straus Family Creamery*
Harmony Hills Dairy	Organic Valley	Stonyfield Farm
Horizon Organic	Radiance Dairy	Wisconsin Organics
Morningland Dairy	Safeway Organic Brand	Woodstock Farms*

Milk Substitutes

YOU CAN BE ASSURED that these milk alternatives don't use GMOs, even if they aren't labeled as organic:

365 Organic Alternative Milks	Nancy's Organic Cultured	Stonyfield Farm O'Soy
Belsoy	Soy*	Tofutti VitaSoy/Nasoya
Coconut Secret*	Organic Valley Soy*	WestSoy
EdenSoy*	Pacific Natural Foods*	WholeSoy*
Imagine Foods/Soy Dream	Silk	Wildwood
Lisanatti	So Delicious	Yves The Good Slice
Nancy's Cultured Soy*	Sun Soy	Zen Don

Eggs

that these egg manufacturers don't use GMOs, even if they aren't labeled as organic:

Egg Innovations Organics
Eggland's Best Organic
Horizon Organic

Land O'Lakes Organic
Nest Fresh Organic
Organic Valley

Pete and Jerry's Organic Eggs
Wilcox Farms Organic

• • • • • • • • • • • • • • • •

Aisle 5: Condiments

that these condiment manufacturers don't use GMOs, even if they aren't labeled as organic:

Annie's Naturals*
Bountiful Bean
Bragg's liquid amino
Carrington Farms Flax Seed
Crofter's Organic
Drew's salad dressing
Eden*
Emerald Cove
Emerald Valley Kitchen
Emperor's Kitchen*
Field Day*

Follow Your Heart*
Ian's Natural Foods
I.M. Health SoyNut Butters
Kettle Brand*
Krazy Ketchup
Maranatha Nut Butters
Miso Master*
Muir Glen, organic ketchup
Nasoya
Newman's Own
Spectrum oils and dressings

SushiSonic Condiments*
The Simple Soyman
Tropical Traditions
Vegan by Nature Buttery
Spread
Vigoa Cuisine
Wholemato
Wildwood
Woodstock Farms*

• • • • • • • • • • • • • • •

Aisle 6: Grains

Cereal

that these cereal manufacturers don't use GMOs, even if they aren't labeled as organic:

Ambrosial Granola
Barbara's, organic
Cascadian Farms
Eden*
EnviroKidz*

Golden Temple
Grandy Oats
Health Valley, organic
Lundberg Rice Cereal*
Nature's Path*

Nonuttin'
Peace Cereal Organic
Ruth's
Simple Sweets
Sunridge Farms

Bread

YOU CAN BE ASSURED that these bread manufacturers don't use GMOs, even if they aren't labeled as organic:

Arrowhead Mills, organic
Bakery on Main
Berlin Natural Bakery*
Bob's Red Mill, organic
Dr. McDougall's Right Foods

Dr Oetker Organics
French Meadow
Natural Ovens Bakery, organic
Nature's Path*

Rudi's Organic Bakery
Rumford Baking Powder
Tumaros*

Pasta, Rice, Beans, Sauces

YOU CAN BE ASSURED that these manufacturers don't use GMOs in their pasta, rice, beans and sauces, even if they aren't labeled as organic:

Amy's
Annie's*
Bob's Red Mill, organic
Casbah (Hain-Celestial)
Dr. McDougall's Right Foods
Eden*
Emerald Valley Kitchen

Fantastic Foods*
Field Day*
Ian's Natural Foods
Lotus Foods
Lundberg Farms Rice
  Sensations*
Muir Glen Organic

Organic Planet*
Rising Moon*
Seeds of Change
Sunridge Farms
TruRoots
Walnut Acres pasta sauce

• • • • • • • • • • • • • • • • •

Aisle 8: Snacks

YOU CAN BE ASSURED that these manufacturers don't use GMOs in their snacks and chocolates, even if they aren't labeled as organic:

Barbara's Organic
Bearitos/Little Bear Organics
Chocolove
Coco Polo
Earthly Treats
Eco-Planet
Eden*
Endangered Species*
Field Day*
Garden of Eatin'
Grandy Oats

Green & Black's Organic
Hain Pure Snax/Hain Pure
  Foods
Health Valley
Ian's Natural Foods
Kettle Brand*
Kopali Organics
Late July Organic Snacks
Lindt Chocolate
Mary's Gone Crackers*
Nature's Path*

Namaste Foods
Newman's Own Organics
Nonuttin'
Peeled Snacks
Plum Organics Tots
Revolution Foods
Ruth's
Simple Sweets
Sunridge Farms
Tasty Brand
Woodstock Farms*

Aisle 9: Beverages

YOU CAN BE ASSURED that these manufacturers don't use GMOs in their juices, energy drinks, cocktail mixes, flavored waters, and other beverages, even if they aren't labeled as organic:

After the Fall
Big Island Organics
Blue Sky
Cascadian Farm
Crofters Organic
Eden*
Field Day*

Frey Vineyards
Mixerz All Natural Cocktail
Mixers
Odwalla
Quinoa Gold
R.W. Knudsen Organic
 (Smucker's)

Santa Cruz Organic
 (Smucker's)
Sea2O Organic Energy Drink
Teeccino Herbal Caffe
Walnut Acres Organic

Appendix Two

Packaging Claims

Here are a few more terms you may find beaming off the labels of your favorite products in the grocery store. They may sound straight-forward, but you may be surprised to learn that they don't always mean what you think!

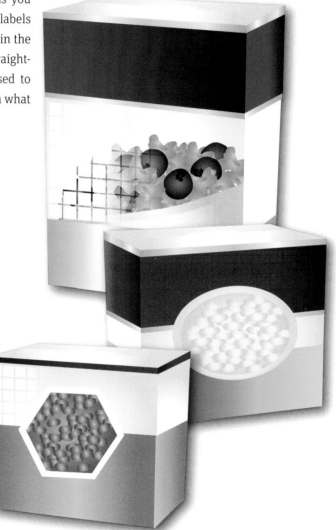

Boasting Added Benefits:

Phrase	What It Means
HIGH IN, RICH IN, OR EXCELLENT SOURCE OF	This means that the food contains 20 percent or more of the average Daily Value (DV) for whatever it's touting. The DV, which is found on the nutrition facts label of all packaged foods, shows us how much of the minimum daily requirement of vitamins, minerals, and nutrients the food is providing. For example, a yogurt advertised as an "excellent source" of calcium contains at least 200 mg of calcium per serving, because the DV for calcium is 1000 mg.
GOOD SOURCE OF	This means the food contains 10–19 percent of the average Daily Value (DV). It is usually on the lower side, since if it were close to the 19 percent, most manufactures would bump it up to get the high, rich, or excellent source designations.
MORE, FORTIFIED, EN-RICHED, ADDED, EXTRA, OR PLUS	These designations can only be used for vitamins, minerals, protein, dietary fiber, and potassium and must contain 10 percent or more of the associated DV per serving.

Light or Low to Downright "No"

CLAIMING A PRODUCT CONTAINS light, reduced, low, no, or is free of a specific ingredient can be tricky. While broccoli is fat-free, you can't legally label a stalk of broccoli as a fat-free food. This is because all broccoli can make this claim. So, only foods that have been specially processed, altered, formulated, or reformulated so as to lower the amount of nutrient in the food, remove the nutrient from the food, or not include the nutrient in the food may bear such a claim (e.g., "low-sodium potato chips").

Phrase	What it means
LIGHT (FAT)	If 50 percent or more of the calories are from fat, fat must be reduced by at least half as compared with the non-fat alternative. If less than 50 percent of the calories are from fat, manufacturers can reduce fat by 50 percent or reduce calories by 33 percent or more per serving.
REDUCED	Can refer to calories, fat, cholesterol, sodium, and sugar. This means at least 25 percent fewer than the average for similar foods.
LOW CALORIE	40 calories or less per 50 g of food or 120 calories or less per 100 g.
LOW FAT	3 g or less per 50 g of food, for meals and main dishes 3 g or less per 100 g and not more than 30 percent of calories.
LOW SATURATED FAT	1 g or less and 15 percent or less of calories from saturated fat, meals and main dishes 1 g or less per 100 g and less than 10 percent of calories.
NO TRANS FATS	Less than .5 g per serving. While this may not seem like a lot, when we eat multiple servings, they add up. Avoid ingredients labeled as *hydrogenated* or *partially hydrogenated,* as these terms indicate trans fats. (To learn about some trans fats that are actually good for you, turn to page 37.)
CALORIE FREE	Less than 5 calories per serving. (Many ready-to-drink beverages contain two or more servings in what looks like a single-serving container—watch out!)
FAT FREE	Less than .5 g per serving, but can contain no ingredient that is a fat or generally understood to contain fat, except if the ingredient has an asterisk that refers to a footnote (e.g., *adds a trivial amount of fat). This is the same for saturated fat.

Phrase	What it means
SUGAR FREE	Less than .5 g per serving, but can contain no ingredient that is a sugar or generally understood to contain sugars, except if the ingredient has an asterisk that refers to a footnote (e.g., *adds a trivial amount of sugar).
CHOLESTEROL FREE	Less than 2 mg per serving, can contain no ingredient that contains cholesterol, except if the ingredient has an asterisk that refers to a footnote (e.g., *adds a trivial amount of cholesterol).
NO SODIUM (SALT) OR SODIUM (SALT) FREE	Less than 5 mg per serving, can contain no ingredient that is sodium chloride or generally understood to contain sodium, except if the ingredient has an asterisk that refers to a footnote (e.g., *adds a trivial amount of sodium).
GLUTEN FREE	Does not contain any of the following: any type of wheat, rye, barley, or crossbreeds of these grains; an ingredient derived from these grains that has not been processed to remove gluten; or, if it has been processed to remove gluten, if it results in the food containing 20 or more parts per million (ppm) gluten, or 20 ppm or more gluten for any reason.

Appendix Three

The Banned Bad Boys

The following Poor Food ingredients are banned in many other developed countries due to their detrimental effects on human health. For numerous suspicious and disturbing reasons, each of these Banned Bad Boys are still allowed in the US food supply. Don't wait for our government to protect you from these dangerous ingredients. Instead, use this list to identify these Poor Food perpetrators on the ingredient list of the foods you are buying. If you see one, don't buy the product. Let's make a statement with our purchasing power—money talks! Leaving Poor Foods on the shelves will speak volumes to the grocery stores and food manufacturers about what informed consumers simply won't tolerate.

Don't remember the specifics on each one of these banned bad boys? Reference their corresponding page numbers to re-familiarize yourself.

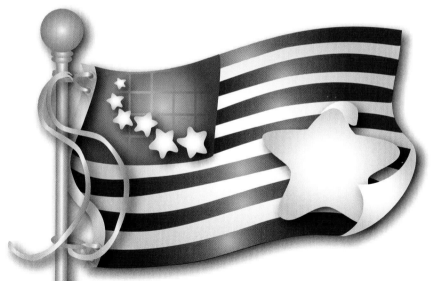

"If the people let government decide what food they eat and what medicines they take, their bodies will soon be in as sorry a state as are the souls of those who live under tyranny."

—Thomas Jefferson, 1781

Counterfeit Colors
(Blue #1, Blue #2, Yellow #5, Yellow #6) • Page 22
. . . found in cake, candy, mac 'n cheese, and medicines

O-No!
(Olestra, aka Olean) • Page 30
. . . found in reduced-fat chips

"Is It In You?" Hope Not!
(Brominated Vegetable Oil aka BVO) • Page 30
. . . found in soda and sports drinks

Crummy Bro-Science
(Potassium Bromate aka Brominated Flour) • Page 31
. . . found in bread crumbs, wraps, rolls, and bagel chips

A-to-Z Bad News
(Azodicarbonamide) • Page 31
. . . found in breads, frozen dinners, and baked goods

The Butylated Brothers
(BHA and BHT) • Page 31
. . . found in gum, nuts, breakfast cereals and meats

Banned for the Bovines
(Synthetic Hormones aka rBGH/ rBST) • Page 32
. . . found in most non-organic milk, cream, and cheese

The Funky Chicken
(Arsenic in Chicken Feed) • Page 97
. . . fed to the majority of non-organic, factory-farmed chickens

Index

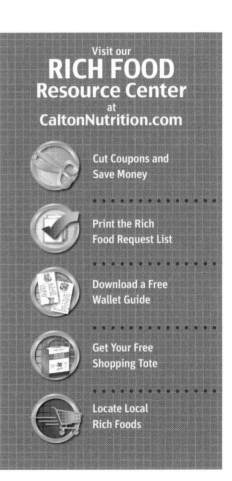

Rich Food, Poor Food Notes

Store: _____

Shopping List

· ·

Rich Food, Poor Food Notes